NOBO
DYTO
LDME

BY HOLLIE MCNISH

Cherry Pie
Papers
Why I Ride

AUDIO

Versus
Hollie and the Metropole Orkest

FEATURED IN

Neu Reekie: #UntitledOne
Bloodaxe Books: Hallelujah for 50ft Women
Bang Said the Gun: Mud Wrestling with Words

NOBO

POETRY AND PARENTHOOD

DYTO

HOLLIE McNISH

LDME

B

BLACKFRIARS

BLACKFRIARS

First published in Great Britain in 2016 by Blackfriars

5 7 9 10 8 6

A CIP catalogue record for this book
is available from the British Library.

ISBN 978-0-349-13435-2

Typeset in Garamond by M Rules
Printed and bound by CPI Group
(UK) Ltd, Croydon, CR0 4YY

Papers used by Blackfriars are from well-managed forests
and other responsible sources.

MIX
Paper from
responsible sources
FSC
www.fsc.org
FSC® C104740

This imprint has no connection with The Order of Preachers (Dominicans)

Blackfriars
An imprint of
Little, Brown Book Group
Carmelite House
50 Victoria Embankment
London EC4Y 0DZ

An Hachette UK Company
www.hachette.co.uk

www.littlebrown.co.uk

This book is dedicated to
Dee and Little One (and Broccoli).

It is an honour to be in this family with you
You are both inspirational in more ways than
you'll probably ever believe.
I love you.

Nobody told me you can't use toilet paper
   Nobody told me that you bleed
   Nobody told me you might need a secret place
   where you can scream.

This is not a collection of polished poems. *Nobody Told Me* is a diary of poems written during the first few years of parenthood. Some of the poems are rushed, some are far too long and still uncut, some were written at four a.m., some on the loo, in hospital, in the car, at work, some were interrupted by cries, screams, laughs ... and some were never really finished. Mostly, they were written on the floor of my Little One's bedroom as she slept.

   All the things I couldn't talk about.

CONTENTS

INTRODUCTION

Glastonbury Festival

I found out I was pregnant on the way to my first Glastonbury Festival poetry gig. In the twenty-minute break between connecting trains from Birmingham to Glastonbury, I decided to face some facts: the fact my boobs were a size larger than ever before; the fact my period still hadn't come; the fact I had been sick every morning, afternoon and evening for the last couple of weeks, making excuses to the women at work for why I had to go and buy another stamp, just to be sick in the local café toilets.

I had an hour to wait at King's Cross Station. I bought two tests and took them into the toilets. Both turned out positive. I went back to the shop, bought one more and got the same result. I washed my hands, got on the train and started to write.

> After King's Cross toilets
> after a blue cross
> after hands-in-face
> with confused then laughing sobs
> I found this spot;
> in the middle of a field
> at the back of a tent
> with no one around.

After the train journey there
three hours staring at three tests
after deciding face to face was best
and despite itching lips
not to phone him yet,
that gave me
three days left.

No one knowing but me.

And I found this horizontal haven
at Glastonbury.

I spent the next three days around the Poetry and Words tent – star-
ing at my stomach, trying not to throw up whilst reciting poems on
the stage and then actually throwing up each morning into a damp,
dew-soaked grass entranceway of a crap one-person pop-up tent. I
also felt deeply guilty; although I hadn't told Dee the news yet, I
felt I needed to tell someone, just in case of an emergency. So the
first other human being to find out that I was pregnant was in fact
a lovely poet called Dreadlockalien; the same man whose van door
I had to bang on in panic at three a.m. the second morning of the
festival, after I woke up covered by a deep pool of muddy, leaking-
tent water.

When I wasn't performing, being sick or sleeping hunched across
the front seat of a renovated van, I just stared, fixated, at families and
gigantic wooden flowers, watching as kids ran around amongst the
jugglers, musicians, acrobats and DJs, wondering how this parenting
thing all worked.

I'd expected a weekend of no-sleep hopes
I'd planned for Dizzee Rascal
DJs, dancing and dope mornings
yawning through sunrise and falling at noon
to new tunes, burnt-out shoes, dance tents
and who's who.

I'd planned to be awake at five a.m.
as shakes of drum'n'bass busted up my head.
instead I lay awake at three a.m.
repeating in my head the word:
'Mum'.
'Mum'.

Alone, in the tent
I heard the hell-bent screams from Trash City slickers
drunken footsteps pass me at sunrise
as my heartbeat quickened
in repetitions:
'Mum'.

So I started a diary there. A diary of all the things I was thinking; all the things I didn't think I was supposed to be thinking; of all the things hidden between the pictures of every pregnancy magazine I picked up, where beautiful pregnant women walk slowly down derelict beaches as pretty flowery dresses drape from their bellies, long (normally straight, blonde, Caucasian) hair blowing gracefully in the breeze. All good. But there are no beaches near me. Most of the pregnant women I meet are too busy trying not to be sick on the commute to work; trying to find old tracksuit trousers that might still fit them; looking after their other kids; or just coming to terms with the speed at

which their entire bodies are changing shape and size and how it feels
for them inside and out.

I started a diary at Glastonbury:

A diary of all the things
I couldn't talk about.

I

PREGNANT

1 month pregnant

Glastonbury was good. This week not so good. But not terrible. I always find it easier to deal with things if I sit outside and look at the stars. Or at least stare at them out of the window. Because they're much bigger than me and the night is cool and I'm tiny and, well, stars make me realise that this sort of stuff, it's just not that fucking important in the grand scheme of the universe. I love the stars for that.

I remember sitting at my window at night after fights at school or broken teenage hearts. Pen in hand, pad of paper, writing poems and staring at the stars, thinking 'Fuck it, it's not so bad.' It's a good place to be, at an open night-time window when everything seems a bit tits-up.

Stood at the sink, hands in the washing-up. It's taken me a day to work out how to do this. This wasn't the moment I'd planned but he's there behind me and it just comes out now – 'I've got to tell you something Dee.'

I breathe in, prepared.

'Me too,' he says.

Smiles. Tensely. Silence.

'You go first then,' I say, glad to have a bit more time to prepare, thinking perhaps he knows already.

'I'm so sorry Hollie, I'm not in love with you any more.'

Lump in my throat. Ah, shit. I'm thinking about the maternity dress I just bought. I'd imagined wearing it at this moment in my life.

Imagined his face kind of excited by the fabric and yellow tones as I broke the news. But I'm in my jeans, hands in the washing-up instead, now not sure if I feel stupid or embarrassed or OK or happy that he's got the guts to just be honest with me. Eyes welling up, either way. Not sure what I should say. But I say the only thing I can.

'I'm pregnant. That's what I had to say. That's quite bad timing, eh?'

We stand in silence. We look at each other. We cry. We swear. We hug. And we laugh too. Because this is shit. But it is almost so ridiculously shit that it is verging on comic. The baby is here to stay, that I know for sure. We both know that immediately. We just have to decide on the rest of it. The practicalities of these two pieces of important news working themselves out together. This is a bit awkward.

I've always begged him to be honest with me. Even if he's just a bit bored or not feeling things the same – just say. Because it's normal life, and I hate the idea of people sticking together when they don't completely want to – then, well, getting old and dying. I don't see the pride in it. I've always begged for honesty. I just didn't expect this now. I feel a bit like I'm in a film, not sure if it's a dark comedy or an overacted drama. Either way, this moment will stick in my mind for a very long time.

So we've spent the evenings this week mainly talking and crying and then sitting in silence. Work has been tricky but a good distraction from a slightly wrenched heart and stomach. Tonight the air is really fresh. I go to the window and open it. Stare at the stars. I cannot complain. I'm twenty-six and I'm healthy. I'm pregnant, which is a magical thing. I'm possibly going through a break-up, but everyone's all right. And if not in love with me any more, he's already in love with this kid. There is still a lot of love here.

If my nurse of a mother has drilled anything into my brain for the last twenty-six years it is that there is a lot of shit going on out there, below the stars. A lot of people are ill. A lot of people are struggling. I am neither. Neither is Dee. Our eyes are a constant sore red and I feel in quite a daze but the stars are still twinkling very brightly. I stare at the sky for a bit, then check for the dress receipt. I'll take it back to the shop tomorrow. I didn't like it much anyhow.

Dress

I feel like my mind has been shaken a bit
I don't really know what to do
for the first time imagining futures
and convincing myself they'd be true

I always thought girls shouldn't indulge too much
in fairytales, rom coms or vows
but I realise I started to do that a little
as soon as the blue cross made out

On a toilet staring wide-eyed and scared
from excitement to panic to glad
and the only thing stopping me weeping out loud
was the thought of him being the dad

Never broody like others, not desperate for kids
I felt sickness out floating to sea
and the only thing stopping the panic attacks
was thinking how happy he'd be

And I didn't want to tell him then
until two more blue crosses had shown
'cos I thought he'd be more disappointed
if I told him and then I was wrong

Two tests later, locked in a toilet,
staring like ghosts at the door
even felt bad at the passion he had
and the thought that he wanted this more

Spent a weekend at Glastonbury, gazing about
adjusting my senses to try
to imagine a life with a child by my side
without fearing I'd not learnt to fly

Not broody like others, desperate for kids,
wondering how I'd make a mum
calming myself with comments he made
imagining me with a bump

I planned walks on pebbled beaches that weekend
I planned the length and style of maternity dress
hand in hand, us, sand on palm,
waves washing the sand from our legs

I imagined the look he might give me
the glint that shook in his eye
I imagined the smile his face would stretch into
as my bump became stretched on all sides

I imagined the tears
he'd be peacefully yelling
the warmth of his hand
pressed onto my belly

Four days alone
I plotted it all –

escaped my urge
to jump up and flee

And all inside my head
his jokes
of breeding
starting three

Of talk of having families
how I'd start at twenty-six
I always said girls shouldn't rose-tint the world
and now I've learnt my bit

Now I'm not really sure what to do
skin colder
mind to rock
and the dress that I thought
would suit this moment
I'll take back to the shop.

1½ months pregnant

All Right

It's gonna be all right
Just a different kind of life
Not burnt or blackened light
'Cos the night still shines as bright
The stars come through the glass still
Silhouettes still pass like ink quills
and though sleep's not quite as still, still
you're here beside me still

And it's gonna be all right
Just a different kind of life
Not comfort picket-fence white
But then I never had that sight
It doesn't mean it's all to shite

We're both here and still alive
And all feelings don't just die
Tripped switch and cold, dark plights
And the air's still in our lungs here

Deep breaths to break the fear
and though tears still fall as fast
now they're paced by heavy laughs

'Cos it's gonna be OK
Just a changed sun dawn new day
Like the interlude is played
second part not quite the same

But it's gonna be OK
Not the standard, boring way
Not fairytales but truth
I'm still thrilled I met with you
And as friends or more or less
I'm still blessed I'm here with you

So let's sweep it up and smile
or pour more mess on the pile
of broken thoughts
and hurting hearts
and just be thankful time is healing ours . . .

I look at the stars and smile. Dee joins me and we cry and laugh a bit
more.

3 months pregnant

We are finally telling people. After twelve weeks of talking and crying and hugging and calmness and decision-making. After twelve weeks of excuses and lies, we can tell people. It's been stranger than I thought. Telling Dee was not how I'd imagined. Telling everyone else hasn't been, either. It's really strange. Embarrassing. Awkward, even. But exciting. Tingly. Scary. Difficult. Really difficult to tell people around us that I'm pregnant.

I am pregnant.

Hello. I am pregnant.

Hello. How you doing? Oh, yeah, by the way, I am pregnant.

Mum guessed ages back, of course. She asked me like ten times already. I hate lying to her.

'Are you sure, Hollie? Your boobs look bigger. Are you sure?'

'No, Mum.'

'Why are you being sick?'

'Hungover, Mum.'

But she's a nurse. I knew she'd know. So I told her first. She was in bed. I walked in, deep breath, and said, 'Oh, by the way Mum, you're right, I'm pregnant.' Then I sprinted out of the room before she could reply, having flashbacks of the day I told her my periods had started and made exactly the same immature but necessary manoeuvre away from any more questioning. She already knew then, as well. I'd been stealing sanitary towels out of her top drawer for over a year.

A lot of my mates guessed too, mainly because I refused a drink at the pub a few times. Said I was on antibiotics. 'Whatever,' Julie said. 'Whatever,' they all said, and let me carry on with the lie, smiling.

My work colleague Emma knew because I stopped having normal tea. She winked and asked me every morning why I had changed my mind about caffeine so suddenly. When I finally admitted she might have a point we laughed in whispers because I was terrified to tell my boss. When I first got the job, my boss made a joke – 'You're not planning a baby, though, are you?' The same jokes appear at the start of new projects – 'As long as you don't get pregnant!'. I understand that it's tricky for business and even more so for small charities like this, but it's not my fault that women might have babies at some point in their life. But I feel bad about it. I shouldn't but I do. My friend said maternity leave was the worst thing that happened to this country. Bah.

How does anyone keep this stuff hidden?

Other people had different reactions:

My boyfriend Dee's mum: ecstatic. That was really, really nice.

My dad: 'My God!' And hugged me. Really tight. He was more excited than I'd expected. He had that cheeky grin on his face that makes him look about thirteen years old.

Phone call to my brother:

'I've got news. Big news.'

'Oh my God,' he also said, 'did you dye your hair pink?'

'What? No. What? I'm pregnant.'

Silence.

'Shit, for real!'

Laughter. I laughed too.

Grandma Number 1:

'Oh love!'

Followed by a sympathetic 'Was it a mistake?'

Followed by 'I thought you were on the pill?'

And a well-meaning but slightly awkward questioning of my contraception arrangements. I was expecting that. I know she's worried about my job. She is also from the generation of women that was made to think pregnancy, a pregnant body especially, was something pretty gross.

Grandma Number 2:

'Is it his?' (After six years with one boyfriend, I'm not sure why this was the first question my gran asked me.)

'Yes, it is Gran.'

'Oh. Do you think you might get married?'

'No, Gran.'

'OK, love.'

Aunties and cousins: all lovely. Smiles and congratulations and 'Don't worry about what people say's'.

Other reactions have been:

Shocked face: '*You?!*'

Both me and Dee have had this in equal measures.

And again:

'*You?!*'

'I can imagine anyone but you two having a baby!'

'I didn't think you wanted kids.'

'I just can't imagine you being a mum!' (I got that one a lot.)

'Amazing!'

'Are you getting married?' No.

'Not even for tax purposes?' No.

'It would be good for your child, to get married – it's not just about you now.'

Other things I'm not writing down because I don't want them in my memory.

And hugs. Nice hugs and awkward hugs and guilty hugs that followed slightly too shocked first reactions.

It wasn't really what I had imagined. I've only seen this stuff happen in films. And I always see it the same. A smart middle-class married couple, usually Caucasian, usually North American, always attractive, wearing clean, white linen shirts have been trying for kids for a while and are finally pregnant. Knowing everyone will be happy about it, they stand holding hands and announce to a room full of eager and excited family: 'We're pregnant' – always 'we'. Everyone is over the moon and everyone cries. The couple look at each other and smile sweet as saccharine.

It wasn't quite like that. But it was still pretty exciting.

5 months pregnant

I'm starting to regret having signed up to these online pregnancy updates – one email every week since week eight telling us what stage of development the baby should be at; telling me what to eat, how to look 'chic' whilst pregnant, and on and on.

Today, the baby should be the size of a large banana, apparently; last month, it was a medium-sized aubergine; the first time I got the update, it was a cherry. I imagined a maraschino stuck on the side of a massive cocktail I cannot drink any more.

I bought a fruit bowl from the market today, thinking it would turn our flat's small kitchen into the sort of cottage where Italian families sit around a big wooden table and share homemade tagliatelle together. I realise not all Italian families do this, or even like tagliatelle, but the ones with large kitchens and wooden tables I imagine might. I used to have a recurrent dream when I was a teenager of a naked baby toddling through vineyards shouting 'Mama, mama' at me. I don't even know if that's the Italian for 'mum'. I think it was after watching repeats of *A Place in the Sun*. Or a Dolmio advert. If I'm honest, it is likely a backlash from my teenage obsession with watching *Stealing Beauty* on repeat from the age of fourteen to sixteen; a film in which a teenage girl loses her virginity in a vineyard by an old tree in Italy. I fucking loved that film. More than was healthy. I wrote heaps of terrible, terrible poems about how I was the last leaf on that olive tree just waiting to be plucked or swept away in the warm Italian breeze. The worst lines I remember are possibly:

I am an ice cube waiting to melt
I'm a flower waiting to be smelt

Basically, I just wanted to shag in a vineyard, but I hid it in bad – and pretty easy to decode – metaphors. I've still never been to Italy. And I now realise the film is as bad as my poems, with one of the worst titles I've ever heard. But back then, for me, it was the shit.

Anyway, I bought the bowl.

The market craftswoman was pregnant too, and when I bought the bowl she cried. Looked me in the eyes and wept.

I thought she was crying because I was her only customer for the day, the week, the month maybe, battling with Habitat factory-made fruit bowls.

But maybe, she was also thinking that day:

Banana Baby

'Your baby should be as big as a banana by now'
'Your sickness may calm down now'
'Your stomach may be sorer now'
'You should feel more tired now'
'You should put on a pound a week now'
'You may be more forgetful now'
'You should think about your finances now'
'You should consider birth classes now'

'You should book your next scan now'
'You should start pelvic exercises now'
'You should clench between each wee now'
'You must clench between each wee now'
'You should get the maternity leave form now
and fill it in and hand it to your boss now'
'You have to tell your boss now'
'You should start thinking about names for the baby now'
'You should decide whether or not you are going to use
disposable or cotton or semi-disposable
or eco-company nappies now'
'You should try to keep the baby happy now'
'You should play the baby classical music now'
'Classical music will make your baby brainy now'
'No Mr Whippy ice-cream now'
'You might have trouble weeing now'
'It may be hard to reach round'
'You should pack your birth bag now'
'You should pack your hospital bag now'
'You should buy sanitary pads now'
'You should buy breast-leak pads now'
'You should buy big pants now,
I mean really, really, really, really big pants now'
'You shouldn't sleep on your back now
or your right-hand side now
and sleep may be uncomfortable now
and you may wake in the night now
and your ribcage may ache now
and your left arm and shoulder blade and leg
may hurt a little now
and you may think about buying
a sculpted pregnant-woman cushion now'

It said:
(discount code below)

'But don't do too much'
'Remember . . . to . . . relax'
'Stress can be very harmful for your baby.'

Maybe she was thinking that.
Your baby should be as big as a banana by now.

5 NOVEMBER

5¼ months pregnant

The midwife visited today. She's a total gem, but fucking obsessed with ice-cream. She keeps talking about it. The particular conversation today went:

Her: 'How are you?' (It's really nice to have someone visit just to ask me this.)

Me: 'Yeah fine, thanks.'

Her: 'Have you remembered the list of no-go foods?'

Me: 'Yep, I've got it.'

She ignores this comment and starts to list them:

'Seafood, certain cheeses, red meat, Mr Whippy ice-cream.'

She stops at this last one, pauses and repeats it:

'No Mr Whippy ice-cream.'

She has already told me this. I know I can't have Mr Whippy ice-cream. I don't get the option that often, anyhow. I tell her 'No problem' again. She then stares deep into my eyes as if she is about to reveal to me why I am on this huge spinning planet and the purpose of bringing another life onto it. She leans in, puts her hand on my shoulder and says:

'Don't worry though, you can have Tesco ice-cream, OK? Any tub, any flavour – chocolate, vanilla, anything. It's only Mr Whippy you can't have. OK? Tesco ice-cream is totally fine.'

It was a moment between us, for sure.

5¼ months pregnant

Today we found out the baby is a girl. I cried. In fear, mainly. I panicked. I don't know why. Now I feel stupid. I'm so embarrassed to even write this down.

Sorry

I don't know why I was feeling so bad
scared that without a wee boy he'd be less want for dad
thoughts coming into my head like acid rain soaking
my brain with stereotypes, bitching and posing.

Lipstick-thin pictures in *Heat* magazine
red circles on blemishes squashing our dreams
I wanted to scream, 'It's a girl! Oh no, please!
This world isn't good enough yet for another she!'

I thought about bleach creams and bullies and beauty
and adverts designed to make girls feel unpretty.
I thought about politics – more dicks than hot dinners –
I thought of a world that makes men likely winners

Until I remembered the people I know
and how none of them fits this same stereotype.

Dee up on stage, I'd imagined a boy there,
rapping son–dad team like Remus and Farma
What a sexist I am! Why am I thinking this shite?
Forgetting Jean Grae, Arianna, Ms Dynamite

Realising the brain-washing media projections
splitting young kids into gendered obsessions.

Forgetting the traumas a young boy can have
forgetting male tears and male heartbreak's as sad
forgetting that boys can have things just as bad
forgetting the girls who hang just with their dads.

Matching tracksuits, I always saw Dee and a son
forgetting a girl can wear just the same one.
For a second I worried about missing out footie
I'd pictured a son and me pass keepy uppies
Forgetting it's *me* who plays in a team
and I'm female
for fuck's sake
and if I had a son
he might hate football too
like my big brother does

What a fuss
I feel sick
I feel stupid and tired

Whether a girl or a boy, the only thing now
is to keep their heart happy and healthy somehow
I feel I've already let my child down
when I should have been nothing but proud.

Sorry Dee. Sorry kid.
I don't know why I thought what I did.

6 months pregnant

Sunrise Sickness

You show me the rainbow inside me.
You force it out of me every day!
Sick on my bike, sick out the car
sick in the office or at the café.

Bright yellow sick in the sink every morning
bright yellow sick and I'm constantly yawning
like the gold at the end of the rainbow, you're calling
and I'm sick and I'm crying as the birds call the dawn in

and when you come out crying
and I pray you will cry
I will try to calm
the screams of mine

and when you come out crying
and I pray you'll be crying
I promise
to show you the rainbows outside.

OK, so I'm trying to be positive but I still feel quite sick. I also can't stop saying 'motherfucker'. I'm trying to stop. I hate the word. But for some reason I have been saying it a lot. In my head, when in public. Out loud, at home. When I wake at five fucking a.m. each morning to be sick. Motherfucker. When I pull over on my bike on my way to work to be sick. Motherfucker. When I pull over at the side of the road in the car to be sick. Motherfucker. When my boobs are sore. When I feel sick again. Motherfucker. Motherfucker. Standing at the end of my bed again at five a.m. feeling miserable, Dee repeating the phrase with me in guilty solidarity.

'Sorry, Hollie. Do you want some ice? Can I do anything?'

I smile, then run to the bathroom to be sick. I try to focus on the positive. I am fine and the baby is fine so far and Dee, well Dee is an absolute legend. Whatever happens, it has been good to be sharing the flat together still. And even though it's gross, the sick is a wee bit fascinating. It's acid sick, the type that people (me, I mean) throw up at parties when they have drunk far too much cheap alcohol, after all their food and drink and insides have been emptied out and all they have left is stomach acid. But somehow my body is keeping the food and drink inside my stomach and only getting rid of the stomach acid. How is that even possible? My body is amazing! And rather than looking like the cold Heinz lentil soup of normal sick, it is a bright, smooth, sun-shine, daffodil yellow. Yeah, just like daffodils, Hollie! Like a rainbow! What am I going on about? It is sick! And it is making me retch louder than I knew humanly possible.

I need to stop swearing. But it helps. More than all the fucking ginger beer in the fucking world. More than nibbling like a goddamn field mouse on a piece of shitty, tasteless dry toast. This is harder than I thought it would be. Sickness and guilt: for swearing so much and for feeling like a fraud. Am I really ready to be a mother? I don't feel like one. A woman last week told me she could feel the spiritual presence of the baby in her womb. *How beautiful*, I thought. *I'm glad you're finding it so fucking enlightening.* I'm just jealous though, I know that. All I feel is sick and scared. The sickness was meant to end months ago. I'm not sure when the fear will end.

Instinct

You can't hear me but I want to say sorry.
I try listening but I can't feel a thing.
They say some women know like an instinct.
I just hope you keep living.
Resting on my bed I feel raindrops splash.
Running through my head with each lightning flash.
One time struck and I'm crying again
hands pressing ice cubes on my stomach.
They melt, thaw on boiling skin.
Swollen breasts too sore to kiss.
My craving hands ache to touch
for affection
but body turns
scared of rejection again.
Dawn wakes up to my head in the toilet
matching the sun shades of acid enjoyment.
Showering pleasures tell me I'm blessed
but I feel too weak to feel it.
Midday flushes, ice cubes again
clinking in glasses and cooling my tongue
hands on my stomach hope you're OK
but I still don't feel very motherly.
I'll be happier if I'm back in love maybe.
Happier when I wake after sunrise.
Happier without my head down the toilet.

Happy when I've seen in your eyes.
Till then I'll smile like I mean it
hoping your dad's lips on mine were for real.
Matching the bile with bright rising sunrays.
Trying to guess how you feel.

I really hope this sickness ends soon. It's rubbish. Working in a tiny office going back and forth between my desk and the toilet making loud noises that everyone can hear. What if I was a teacher? What did my mum do in the surgery when she was pregnant? 'Please excuse me, I'll be back in a minute to do your smear test, madam, I just need to vomit for the five-millionth time this morning.' At least my job isn't with any members of the public. At least I'm not trying not to gag *and* do smear tests at the same time. Or on a perfume counter. Or handling food. So many jobs that would be terrible to be pregnant at. Four people in the office. I should be bloody grateful. It's really fucking hard working when you're pregnant. I didn't realise it would be.

6½ months pregnant

My belly is still so hot. The ice cubes that I'm rubbing on it are now melting in approximately ten seconds flat, quicker than the refill and freezing process can possibly keep up with. I'm glad I'm pregnant in winter. So glad for the cold air. For the frost. What I'm less glad about now is all the advice I'm being given based on these ice cravings.

Since the start of my pregnancy, my cravings have been a pretty hot topic. I imagined peanut butter and gherkins, both things I love. But most people around me had other advice:

Meat

You should eat meat.
You need to eat meat.
It's really important now to eat meat.
You can't have a healthy baby if you don't eat meat.
You'll get cravings for meat.
I bet you'll crave meat.
meat
meat
meat

fucking meat

meat.

Nearly seven months in and I still have no cravings for meat. My mum says I don't need to eat meat, and she's a nurse. My gran says I do.

But I only want ice; to put it in my mouth and rub it on my hot, stretched belly skin, over my forehead and in every drink I order. I look like a weirdo but I do not give a toss any more. I can't do that with a lump of meat. I can't go to my friend Anna's fancy fridge, press a button and have a glass full of cool, crushed meat to refresh me.

Still, the conversations carry on:

Them: 'Are you craving meat yet?'

Me: 'No.'

Them: 'Are you craving meat yet?'

Me: 'No. But the doctors say the baby is healthy so don't worry.'

Them: 'Are you craving meat yet?'

Me: 'No, just ice.'

I shouldn't have admitted this last bit to anyone, because now all I'm getting is:

I think you might be anaemic.

Craving ice can mean you have an iron deficiency.

You need to eat meat.

Meat is full of iron.

You need meat.

meat

meat

meat

fucking meat

meat.

I can't count how many times I've been told this in my life. I turned veggie at four years old, according to my family. For two weeks, my brother supposedly set the farm toys up for me to look at, then told me exactly which of my favourites I was eating – at one point squirting a McDonald's Happy Meal toy fish, flounder, at me as I munched on a fish-finger sandwich. I cried, and never ate meat or fish again. Nothing against it, I was just traumatised. My brother was vegetarian for a good month before re-succumbing to Ronald McDonald's charms.

My mum lied to me for a couple of years, feeding me 'vegetarian mince' and 'mushroom sausages', but then felt bad and gave in to my refusal to eat 'my farmyard toys'.

In fairness, it definitely increased my popularity at school, as people learnt that going to McDonald's with me meant that they'd get a free extra burger, as I took out the meat from mine and stuffed the sweet, gherkinned sugary bun full of fries instead. Anyway, people have worried ever since about this non-meat-eating problem. Everyone else in my family eats meat. I've been told loads of times I must be anaemic, by family and friends alike. So I've checked loads of times. I'm not. I never have been.

But this meat love sticks. It's a strong opinion based, I think, on health recommendations made by people with a massive stake in the industry. And now that I'm pregnant the meat love has really turned up a notch. Now guilt is added:

> *I know you don't eat it normally Hollie*
> *but it's not just yourself*
> *it's your child you're endangering.*
> *When you're pregnant, you just have to be extra careful.*
> *It's not about you any more.*
> *It's about the baby.*
> meat
> meat

meat
guilty meat
meat.

Dee doesn't eat meat either. Just fish. The best comment he got went like this:

Friend: 'Hollie's pregnant?'

Dee: 'Yeah.'

Friend: 'Did you start eating meat then?'

Dee: 'No.'

Friend: 'How did you get her pregnant then?'

So I'm anaemic and he's unable to produce sperm. All down to a lack of meat.

Don't get me wrong, some meat *is* a good source of iron. And iron is important, in life generally as well as in pregnancy. And eating ice *can* be a sign of anaemia. I'm not knocking that.

So I did another iron test today. Turns out, I'm not iron-deficient.

So I will keep crunching ice and sticking it down my T-shirt everywhere I go till it melts in beautiful trickles along my belly. And while it is running down my skin easing my sickness, I will sing:

Ice
ice
fucking
ice
ice

to anyone else who tells me the baby needs meat.

6½ months pregnant

I keep getting little shakes of excitement. Tremors inside my body, building up. I am actually pregnant. I have told everyone now and I am slowly starting to believe it myself. I'm not imagining it. I bought a flowery maternity dress today on my lunch break. Took it home, tried it on, for a minute imagined myself walking down a beach in it, then realised it was just an advert knocking around in my head, and took it off. I took it back to the shop the next day. It just wasn't right. But for a second, I had felt a bit like it was a possibility again.

I worry a lot about these expectations. But in between the worry and pain and sickness and panic, when everyone else is away, when everyone else shuts the hell up, there are definitely little frissons of excitement sparking in my veins, making me feel a little bit special. Like something special is happening. Like when my mum used to tell me I'd grow an apple tree in my body if I ate the seeds and I used to dream about the branches slowly taking shape and growing from my fingers into huge, shiny, red, juicy apples, my hair made of leaves, my body stretching to the skies above a huge forest. For some reason I never thought about the fact that if that did happen, the apple tree would slowly push through my internal organs and skin and maim me as it stretched until I was a heap of broken bones and ripped flesh.

I read *James and the Giant Peach* again recently. I know it's a kids book but I am in still love with Roald Dahl. Rereading that moment after the mysterious man gives James the magic bag that will change his life, and he stumbles and drops it and all the green worm-like seeds dart into the ground, and James is so scared and sad but then the next day he sees that huge, beautiful peach hanging from the tree's branch, bent over with the weight, overshadowing the misery of life with Aunt Sponge and Aunt Spiker. I imagine that peach, the flesh and the juices inside and the magnificence it created in that derelict garden. But most of all that feeling of magic, that something in the ground is stirring and you have no idea where it will take you or what it means but you just know that there is magic in it.

That's how I feel sometimes about this. Like this baby is going to fly with me on a gigantic juicy peach powered by thousands of squawking seagulls over the ocean – like there is life growing inside my body. Right now. Inside my flesh.

23 DECEMBER

7 months pregnant

I am seven months pregnant. My belly is getting pretty big. My grandma sent me a cardie in the post last week with a note that it might help me 'cover up the bump, love'.

'Do you realise how funny you look?'

The work Christmas party was crap.

'Do you realise how funny you look?'

I am now counting up the number of times people have asked me this sort of question. Most often followed by:

'It's just so strange to see your body like that, Hollie!'

It clocked up a lot at the work Christmas party, followed by uninvited drunken hands placed on my belly. Why are you doing that? You didn't touch my belly before – don't touch it now. I think I'm overreacting. It's probably quite a sweet thing: curiosity. And it's awkward handing out the yeses and the noes. *You can touch my belly. No, not you, get the fuck off.* A 'People Who Have the Right to Touch My Bump' list. A bit divisive, maybe! But the party was too much. I clocked about five minutes in total where someone's sweaty, drunken hand wasn't rubbing, patting or simply perching on my hot, stretched skin.

Maybe I'm just moody because once again everyone is drunk, staring at me, and I am the sober pregnant person feeling stared at and clutching a soft drink. I really appreciate the thought but lemonade in a wine glass is getting a bit tiring now. I just drink water and save the cash. It's harder than I thought to be the sober one at a party. It's even harder to be the sober pregnant one.

Do you realise how funny you look?

Christmas in Scotland with the family. I love it. Being the only English-accented family member, it's like my ears are really home, lying in a warm bath of Glasgow and Stirling voices. The first day there, we plan lunch at Dobbie's, the local garden centre. As we get up to leave, Gran asks me if I want to borrow her ring.

'No thanks,' I say, smiling, trying to brush it off.

She asks again.

I say, 'I don't want to borrow the ring thanks, Gran.'

She says, 'I thought you liked wearing jewellery?'

I know it's a caring thing and she's trying to be subtle but it's not working.

I say, 'It's all right Gran.'

She says she just doesn't want me to get hurt.

> 'Here's a cardie, love –
> hide the bump'
> 'It's a baby,' I say
> She smiles and looks away
> Today we're off for lunch
> so my Grandma takes her glove off
> and offers me her ring to wear
> and though I feel a little shamed
> I know she's just protecting me
> from how people would've been to her
> if she had done the same.
> The other Grandma takes my waist
> and holds it tighter than a glove.
> 'Loads of my generation got knocked up too,'

she whispers,
'we just kept it covered up
and married bloody quickly.'

Unmarried and pregnant, I realise that is what my body now stands for.

I can't imagine how it was for my grandmas back then because, right now, I'm so hurt to think that I'm in any way an embarrassment to the family because I have a child inside me. A healthy child. I realise my body now tells the world: I, Hollie McNish, have had unprotected sex. Men's bodies don't give those facts away. Anyway, no one's bothered about men having sex. No one has asked Dee if he wants to wear a ring when we go out. Or even if he's planning to get married. And no one dares ask him the questions I get, like 'I thought she was on the pill?' or 'Did you not put a condom on your penis?' or 'Was it planned?' – which basically amounts to the same question – they just ask me, as if being visibly pregnant allows you some right to ask about my sex life all of a sudden. Anything else you'd like to know while we're on the topic, anyone? What position we did it in? What underwear I was wearing at the time? Was I fooled into believing the withdrawal method would work? Anything else?!

Dee's just standing and laughing quietly behind me and purposefully rubbing my belly and saying how much he loves the massive bump. My gran is smiling, but cringing a little and telling him to stop. I just wanted to go out for lunch. Eat a jacket potato, side of coleslaw, drink a cup of tea. I don't want to be a circus freak. Still, I wrap the cardie round my belly, imagining how horrible it must've been for my grandmas when they were pregnant – that feeling that you've done something wrong and that everyone can now see the evidence.

Do you realise how funny you look?

Someone shouted 'Teen mum!' at me in the street the other day. I shouted back, 'I'm twenty-six!' I wish I hadn't. I work with a lot of teen mums and I see how brave they are and what they go through every day, despite what the Vicky Pollard stereotype might suggest. God knows how they feel when they're treated like that. I should've just said, 'Yes. I am.' Damn, what an idiot. They're the current generation's scapegoat for pregnancy shaming.

Do you realise how funny you look?

So, yes, I am unmarried and sexually active. Unmarried and we didn't wear a condom. And I am given a cardigan and a pretend wedding ring to ease the shame for everyone. OK, not everyone, not most people – this is a different generation, I know – but it still feels hard. I tell myself to listen to the majority, the ones who are excited, who smile when I tell them, who hug me. Who want to touch my belly. Maybe that's a good thing, then. Maybe wanting to touch my belly is a good thing. It's worse when they don't want to, I guess. What if nobody wanted to?

Do you realise how funny you look?

And other similar phrases. I note them all down now.

The List: What Not to Say to a Pregnant Woman

Do you realise how funny you look?
Have you looked at yourself in the mirror?
It's just that it's so strange to look at your figure
It's just that it's just so much bigger.
Are you sure it's not twins?
You look bigger to me
Than you should, than you see on those soaps on TV!
As they wrap their arms round and stare at my body
Do you realise you just look so goddamn funny?
Do you realise I've never imagined you fat
And when I see your physique I just can't believe that.
I wouldn't call it a miracle, she said,

It just looks quite strange
With your thin arms and legs but a mid rearranged.
They say:
Do you realise what you look like?
And when you waddle the street!
Can you sleep sound at night?
Joking how it makes them feel better to see me look shite
Bigger than them for the first time in my life.
And I smile, and I laugh, reply once or twice
But honestly, those comments are not very nice.
When in a short space of time you lose what you knew
The size and the shape and the feel that was you
Coming to terms with becoming a mum
Or just coming to terms with treating a bump
With a baby inside, feeling limbs long and kicking
From anxious, magical, scared shitless and livid
Passing by mirrors having forgotten the truth
Then reminded in silhouettes of stomach balloons
Insecure, unsure about what you're going to do
And the last thing you want is people staring at you
A central attraction on every street march
People stare on the bus, on the train, in the park
Heads tilt sympathetically assuming 'mistake'
Two shouts of 'Teen mum!' and it's ruined my day.
Desperate to welcome this change as amazing
To walk the streets proud with big belly blazing
To soak up the strangeness in wonder and awe
And calmly enjoy this new opening door
But more
I wanna run hide and rest in the dark
No light, so no eyes to run over the scars
No smart passers-by not giving up seats

No friends making jokes that they're 'thinner' than me
Some days I want to run, hide and stay in the dark
No visual body, no funny remarks
'Cos some days I feel sick that there's growing inside me.
Next day I'm overjoyed at life showing inside me
And the timing is crucial 'cos on days feeling shit
When my body's a pod and I can't move my hips
Those are the times I feel sunk, lined and hooked
When you ask if I realise how funny I look.

I just smile, maybe laugh, but in my head my heart's blue
Thinking *Yes, of course*
I fucking well do.

25 DECEMBER

7 months pregnant

It is Christmas Day and I am surrounded by presents for a baby not even born yet. My family is so lovely. So thoughtful. The floor looks like a multicoloured grotto. I feel really guilty.

I feel guilty because we have been lying to everyone since the scan. And today, as I open a pile of beautiful baby clothes, everyone is discussing the lie.

This is the lie:

Them: 'Is it a boy or a girl?'

Us: 'Oh, we didn't want to find out.'

I hate lying but I am not telling anyone that we do know. Because I live in a strange country called the UK where, for some reason, shops only use one colour for small humans with a fanny and one colour for small humans with a willy. Do they save money if they buy the dye in bulk? It must be that. I can't see any other reason for this weird obsession. I don't hate light pink, I just didn't want that to be the only colour in the flat or the main colour my baby sees as she works out the world and her place in it.

Her: 'Who am I? What is this planet? What am I doing here?'

Us: 'You are light pink. You like princesses, butterflies or flower logos on all your clothes. You don't like trains or robots or tractors.'

So we say: 'We didn't want to find out.'

This has annoyed people more than I thought. Lots of people

42

have said they won't know what colour to buy baby clothes in.

I feel like saying: If you do want to buy baby clothes, and I'm really, really grateful if you do, here are some colour ideas:

Red
Orange
Yellow
Green
Blue
Indigo
Violet
Black
Brown
White
Cream
Turquoise

When did we forget the existence of other colours? I know the shops are full of pink and blue, so if there aren't other colours just choose either, I say. I like both of those colours and I don't care if people think my baby is a boy or girl. Babies all look the same anyway and I'm pretty sure there is no scientific evidence that a baby boy dressed in light red will morph into a monster. Or that baby girls in light blue will explode. For my more homophobic friends, I also don't think there's any evidence that a certain shade of a certain colour wrapped around a baby's skin will soak through into their blood and brain and affect whether they fancy men or women or both as they grow up. Saying that, I'm pretty sure if you dress a baby in red it will grow up voting Labour. Or supporting Arsenal.

Anyway, for now, we don't know the sex. Ask me another question please. Because I hate lying. It's horrible. Sorry, everyone.

7½ months pregnant

For Christmas, Mum bought me another ice tray. Dee has been struggling with the turnaround time of refilling just one ice tray when my cravings strike. So she got us another. Safe.

I have also just finished *Half the Sky* – stories about women from all over the world. Another Christmas present from Mum. 'Childbirth is the biggest killer of women worldwide,' I read. Thanks Mum, good choice right now. Did you realise I'm pregnant? Just the ice tray would've been fine!

I keep reading it, though. And this one story, I read over and over. Make a cup of tea and read it again. I cannot get it out of my mind. I will stop complaining about my morning, day and night sickness; about people touching my belly; about fizzy soft drinks at parties; about whether I feel sexy or not. It's really nothing. The woman in the story is my age, and pregnant. I went shopping with my mum today and when she asked what I was thinking I read her this poem. She said it spoilt her first grandma shopping experience and why couldn't I just say 'Baby blankets'? I said she was the one who gave me the book.

Hollow

We started quite similar, two young girls 'knocked up'
Boyfriends excited and mums and dads chuffed

Our friends buzzing by to put hands on our bumps
Both belly and boobs getting shockingly stump.

We started quite similar, both bellies slow-rising
Two plum-ripe tomatoes grow stretch marks in lines
While we're both walking home after work in the office
We try not to waddle as passers-by's eyes are on us.

We started quite similar, both woken at dawn
To two kicks in the pelvis, both giggle and yawn
Now she lies at the side of the road simply screaming
I'm home, she just groans, both our feet up, hers bleeding

'Cos there's no march going on in my city you see
No war, so that war crime's not used against me
I might walk the streets hunchbacked, but baby lies safely
And whilst mine may be ice, it's revenge that she's craving.

So when you ask what I'm thinking, is it boots, cots or
            mittens?
Truth is, I'm just thankful it's here that I'm living

'Cos as my stomach bulges like a water balloon
Her hollowed-out body lies like a carcass consumed
In the wrong time, the wrong street, the wrong country or place
On the wrong side or the wrong tribe, the wrong party or race

Both trying not to waddle as passers-by's eyes all watched,
But whilst mine passed me by, hers circled and stopped.

Radio announcements as troops told to target
'Mothers, children, unborn Moses baskets'

With knives and machetes like cutting through ham
They slice round her belly to remove what they can.

We started quite similar, two young girls 'knocked up'
My boyfriend excited, hers hung himself up.
My mum and dad chuffed, her mum and dad mourning
And as flies buzz her belly, my friends' hands still swarming

'Cos there's no war going on in my city you see
No radio orders to ethnically cleanse me
So when you ask what I'm thinking with a baby inside me
My hands clasp the skin tight and my mind runs in hiding

So when you ask what I'm thinking, Babygros, toys or clothes?
I just smile and nod 'cos truth is, I don't know

So when you ask what I'm thinking every time that it kicks
Ask what I think when its heart beats so quick
The thing I think most, though it might sound quite sick
Is *How the fuck could you cope if they cut out your kid?*

But there's no war going on in my city you see
So that war crime's not used as a weapon against me
No knife waiting bluntly to cut through my womb
As her body lies clutching a hollowed-out tomb

The thing I think most, and it's making me sick
Is *How the fuck could you cope if they cut out your kid?*

9 JANUARY

7½ months pregnant

The kicks are going nuts now. I have an ambidextrous footballer inside my body. The first kicks were fluttering. Now, it's unbelievable. A group of fourteen-year-old students in the front row of a poetry assembly I did last week nearly fell off their seats screaming as a satsuma-sized foot shape made its way stretching the skin out of the side of my stomach. It was a serious poem, I couldn't understand why they started screaming. I feel like Sigourney Weaver in *Alien*. I can't help poking the foot or the fist a little when it shoots out. I'm starting to love this. I find myself staring for hours at my stomach. My hand, Dee's hand, friends' hands, all waiting, staring at it like the new TV in the room. Then the screams:

'Oh my God, did you feel that!'

'Damn! I missed it.'

It's weird. No. It's amazing. So amazing. It's an honour to have this experience.

'Sorry, Dee,' I say. He puts his hand on my belly and smiles. The baby kicks his palm. Left-winger, then.

Kick Me

I know it might sound strange to others
but I like it when you kick me.

It's like when I feel that pain
I know you're right here with me
and baby even though it hurts quite deep inside me
when I feel your fist or kick rough by my skin, it's like
I know you're there right by me.

My friends look disgusted, staring at the patches
on my stomach, side or ribcage
they say they've seen you at it

and though it hurts a little at the time
my breaths remain like bating
I find my hands rubbing the sideline stripes
but my mind in constant waiting

for the next body contact
and more and more
it's less frustrating
at first it made my stomach lurch
but then I'd miss the thrill sensation
and now

I wait
between each kick of yours
I count the clock
with each hand tick for yours
pray I feel a punch or elbow flick
to prove your heart's still quick for more
'cos sometimes that's the only proof
that you're still there and I'm still due.
The only proof for dad and me
that you're still there, alive,

'cos we can't see you
so we wait.

Breathe in.
Hands on my belly.
Swollen stomachs knotted sick.

Until we feel those tiny feet of yours again.
Baby we love it when you kick.

12 JANUARY

7½ months pregnant

Oh my God, last night was nuts. Jokes. Bit gross in fact.

So, I go to a club. Pretty pregnant, but Dee was emceeing there and Taskforce were on the line-up and I really wanted to see them. I also knew there was a soft leather couch in the middle of the club in front of the stage, and that it was a smallish venue in Peterborough, close enough to get home quickly after. So I decided to go.

I was ready for the normal annoying things that happen when I've been out to gigs whilst pregnant. Comments like:

'Should you really be out?'

'Is that OK in your state?'

'What about the loud music?'

'I hope you're not drinking?'

Or when you go to a party and someone immediately gets you a soft drink without even asking what you want.

But last night was not that.

We get in the club. It's a bit grotty but the music's great and I like the dark, dingy, sweaty feel of places like this. I go get a drink and flop onto the couch to watch the bands. The tired leather and the cold of the fabric feel great on my back. Dee has to go backstage. My belly is bulging over the top of my stretchy leggings and I feel pretty tired but still, it's good to be out. Even if I am sitting on my own – stone-cold sober. I like the music enough.

A woman spots me straight off and rushes over, pilled up and extra-friendly. 'You're pregnant! Fuck! Cool!' she starts. 'I was pregnant!' And sits down next to me.

'I've got two kids at home, with their dad. My mate's just had a baby. I'm out with her husband. I mean, not like that, well, not really. Not shagging. Well, it's just that she's got a newborn and you know, that can kill the passion a bit, you know. And me and my husband are done. I'm not cheating – we're not doing anything. Just want a few drinks and well, maybe, you know. What's your name?'

We chat for a bit about her non-affair with her mate's husband and about how babies lead folk to stray away. She's pretty funny and for the first time absolutely and totally positive about me being pregnant. It's a relief. She goes off to dance with the guy, walking across the sticky dance floor just as another woman slips on her stilettos and goes tits-up, sliding across the wooden floorboards dragging her man with her. Everyone pisses themselves laughing, then carries on dancing, groping and head-nodding.

It's funny being sober here, I feel like some sort of reporter. A spy. I watch people dance and lech and grind down and imagine how long before I'm gonna be making a drunken tit out of myself again. It's been a long time since that happened.

About half an hour later, I'm just chilling out listening to the music when a guy walks towards me. He looks about seventeen. He sits down next to me, licks his lips a bit and says 'All right?' with a simultaneous flirty eyebrow-raising. 'I'm all right yeah,' I say. 'Yeah, you look all right,' he replies. He's pretty pissed, but still, I assume he's not seen the massive bump. 'Yeah, I look pregnant,' I say, smiling, thinking that for once this being-pregnant thing is gonna work to my advantage. But no, it has the opposite effect. He replies, 'Yeah,' and licking his lips again slower this time, 'I can see.' Licking his fucking lips! I tell him I just wanna hear the music and can he leave me alone? So he does. Dee comes over to check I'm all right. I am all right. He starts his set.

Then, about fifteen minutes later, it happens again. With a different, older guy. 'You pregnant, yeah?' he starts, looking me up and down, but mainly down. Not my face he's into, I'm sure of that. This one's harder to shift and keeps asking about what month of pregnancy I'm in, in a tone that mimics the voice I imagine he'd put on to ask what pants I'd like to wear when we get back to his steaming love pad. What the fuck? I look at him in stunned silence, try to hide my laughter, then after a bit too close manoeuvring, I start talking about my boyfriend and point-ing him out. Finally, he walks off bored, and I get to listen and chill out.

I'm not one to think that any guy who comes over and chats to me is chatting me up. I don't get it a lot at all. But these were definitely lip-licking, sexually motivated, winking moves.

I also understand there are people who find the pregnant body sexy; that there are women who find being pregnant very sexy too. I've read about them in magazines. I guess it's just that I don't. I really don't. In fact, the idea of having sex this heavily pregnant is really not in any way a turn-on for me. Just putting it out there. Even in the supposed comfort of doggy style. It always feels a little odd. Maybe just 'cos I feel a little odd.

The next day, I phone my mum to tell her how the night was. I tell her about the guys. She immediately, not a second to ponder on it, says:

'They were probably thinking that if they got their leg over at least they knew they couldn't get you pregnant.'

God, that might be it. Nice, Mum – nice.

8 months pregnant

I promised I wouldn't moan and I know it's not a big deal but I need to vent. I stood up on the Tube for nearly an hour today, from Balham to King's Cross. Northern line with minor delays, and no one offered me their seat. I'm not built for this.

Poetry gigs are always taking me to London just to remind me why I love the fact I do not live in this shitty city. Maybe it's my fault for taking gigs so late on in pregnancy. I am eight months pregnant, my belly bulging like a water balloon and no one gives me their seat. A few disapproving looks, maybe it's all in my head, but I'm sure they are disapproving. Some tuts. Tuts at an unborn baby.

A few nervous glances quickly flicking back to Kindles and I wonder if they're all reading porn now you can't see the covers. I'm sure that lady is. My belly is sore, my hips are sore, not today please. Pregnancy makes you stand out: it does not provide you with the confidence to waddle up to a total stranger who has purposely not moved from their seat to say, with the whole carriage watching, 'Erm, excuse me, would you mind if I sat there and you stood up, because as you might be able to tell I have a baby in my belly and it's pretty fucking heavy right now.'

Or something more polite. Some of my other friends are more bolshie. No, 'bolshie' is a bad word. More confident. There are badges, they say, you can get from London Underground that say 'I'm pregnant' so that everyone is sure of it, but I'm not sure of this. At eight weeks maybe – when you feel sick and light headed but have no real physical clues for others to go by. Not at eight months – it's pretty damn obvious and I don't like living in a world where this is necessary. For sure, it isn't always needed. People do stand up. But not today.

So I stand, holding the bottom of my belly to take some of the weight off the shooting pains in my back and stare at this one man. He looks in his thirties, healthy, fit, fresh-faced, slightly arrogant, suited, shining-black patent shoes, and then his gaze meets mine. He has definitely seen me. I smile, that weak smile like a pathetic sigh and lower my eyes. He's seated on the seats with the sign behind that this place is for people like me. People like *me*, you fucking idiot. (I don't say that.) Or elderly people. Or anyone that can't stand easily or for long. I know my friend would walk straight up, her belly beaming like a warning light, and ask him to get up, but in my head I go through all the things that might be up with him, all the illnesses he could have that make it hard for him to stand up too, and how embarrassing if I ask him and he tells me he can't stand. He has definitely seen me. He has looked at my belly. Of course he'd stand up if he could. *He might have bad knees*, I think, *might have had an operation last week, bladder issues or any other problems I can't see.* So I stand, feeling like the heaviness of my bowling-ball belly pushing on my bladder might make me wee my pants right there, staring into space, trying not to hate humankind, and finally we're there. King's Cross.

The guy stands up and walks across me, out of the Tube, and sprints down the platform to catch his train. There was nothing wrong with his legs. He just didn't want to give his seat up. Too important, I guess.

Git.

I hate London. I hate doing gigs. I hate poetry. I hate being pregnant. I hate being such a fool. I want to go home. I have never been so tired in my life. I just wanted to sit down. Why do I feel like I've done something wrong? I'm allowed to be pregnant, aren't I?

9 FEBRUARY

8½ months pregnant

Is she trying to drag the earth right inside me?
Is she trying to feel the wind and the rain?
It's like she's heard what we've said
– less than one month still left –
and she's desperate to come out and play.

I finished my day job yesterday. I no longer have to ride my bike half an hour to the office with my belly resting on the centre frame. Although cycling is much easier than walking. Walking is tricky now. So is wiping my bum, sleeping, standing, rolling from one side of my body to the other – especially at night – looking at my toes or my fanny, and breathing. In fact, everything is quite difficult, except kneeling on all fours watching films or reading in a non-sexual doggy position and waiting for a baby to come out of my body. I don't have the urge to clean my house or 'nest' as it's called in the email updates I am for some unknown reason still reading. Our baby is now a marrow, the size that would win gardening competitions in small villages. All I want to do is eat ice. And it is snowing. I am so happy it is snowing. This week I have eaten two pint glasses of snow, got through fifteen ice-cube trays, refilled madly by Dee. It's all about the ice. Ice and dirt now. Good, cheap cravings.

Ice and Dirty Potatoes

Is she trying to drag the earth right inside me?
Is she trying to feel the wind and the rain?
It's like she's heard what we've said
– less than one month still left –
and she's desperate to come out and play.

'Cos that's the only real explanation
I can think for these feelings I've grown
now with each day she gets larger
these cravings get harder
as I battle the ice formed on snow.

My colleagues list theirs like a trophy
say they ate more chocolate than ever before
but for me the one vice is large chunks of ice
dripping frozen cold drops to my throat.

Now my mouth sings out for the feeling
of frost on my lips and my tongue
and in the snow-covered hilltops
of Gran's Scotland road
I see dinner, breakfast and lunch.

Crunching ice of hardened snow in my teeth
a relief like never before.
From the crunch of each break
now crushed, my mind shakes,
and I pray there's no sunshine or thaw.

I gnaw ice lollies, icicles, ice cubes and slush
and breathe deep on my bike for an icy-cold rush
till my lungs feel the chill of the air and fill up
with a freshness that brings me to new forms of love.

I love crunching it, sucking it, melting it out
till the ice-cube rack's empty and lollies run out
and from the depths of my stomach I'm sure she's about –
was too hot in that womb
now feet up
chilling out.

An igloo-bred baby, snuggling up
with my tongue on the snowflakes, cupping it up
like an addict fulfilled, there's a new sort of love
when you pass me a drink with ice in the cup.

I choose cafés based on their ice game now. Hollow is best. Rounded
not square. Slightly soft. Matt white, not see-through. Crumbly. Even
better are those crushed ice buttons like on my mate Anna's swanky
fridge. I think she's getting suspicious about how often I visit now. But
the ice is amazing. She is too, I mean. It's not just for the ice. She's bril-
liant. Add a bit of water, leave it to melt a little. Perfect. Or the Slush
Puppies that I used to get when I was fourteen on dates with Chris or
Thurston at the local bowling alley and arcades. I'm obsessed with ice,
the smell of dirty potatoes and mouldy crumbling bricks. When we go
out, Dee immediately gets me a 'Tap water with loads and loads of ice
in a wine glass, please.'
    'Yeah, yeah, she's pregnant' – I've heard him say a few times now.

Once, the smell of perfume thrilled me
my boyfriend's scent sexy and fresh.

now it's damp wetted earth, mould, tree bark and dirt
and the tingle runs through to my chest.

I walk close to mud and inhale
and feel every lung muscle cramp
and in my friend Maddy's flat
like heaven's doormat
I sat sniffing the corners of damp.

It's like being so horny and having no way to fulfil it
I feel I can't breathe as deep as I'm wishing
as my nostrils dilate and my breath becomes livid
my lungs cry for more, expand to new limits.

Breathing market potatoes root-deep in soil
I sit sniffing their skins as the pan overboils
I want the grit through my fingers of dewy, cold earth
I want to breathe in the secrets and pieces of dirt.

I yearn for the scent of the bricks in the garage
dig a home in the soil, now I'm envying rabbits
and on an underground tour of Edinburgh's vaults
I could've stayed in the cellars just smelling the mould.

I've told my friends I'm moving into a tree
surrounded by earth, ice cubes and freeze
and somewhere I'm sure she's resting inside
with the smells of this world and the cool of the ice
as if she's heard what we said
– Less than one month till birth –
so she's dragging the earth from outside me to her.

Desperate to sense it, she giggles these cravings
as I sit crunching ice and sniffing dirt on the pavements.

When no one is watching, I cup up the snow and shovel it into my mouth. When no one is watching, I sniff the earth, lick stones and stare into drilled holes in the ground where workmen are digging. When no one else is watching, I don't feel like a freak; a freak with swollen boobs, a bulging heavy belly and snow melting down my chin. When no one is watching, I feel amazing. Like that gigantic, ripe, juicy, magic peach. When I'm alone this is all so amazing. I am fascinated by it; by the cravings, by my body, by you. Why are we not more fascinated by this stuff?

You inside. Can you hear me? When your dad sings to you, can you hear him? When he rubs my belly and stares through the skin as if he has X-ray vision? Now that work is finished for a while and I get to sit by myself and actually take this in – take you in – I realise I already have a baby living beneath my flesh who I will meet soon. A stranger inside my body. I am not Sigourney Weaver in *Alien*, I am a real-life Russian doll. I eat another handful of snow, first clenching it in my fist so it is verging on the solid ice of the snowballs you got a detention for throwing in school.

Two weeks seems far away. I look at my belly. A fist punches through the skin and I touch it. I'm holding hands with a stranger who has lived inside me for nearly nine months. I hope you can hear me. You are a snow baby, making me eat snow and ice like my life is dependent on it.

15 FEBRUARY

8¾ months pregnant

Today is a good day. I can chat to you properly. I took you to my favourite spot today and stared out over the water. Finally everything is quiet. The water. The ducks. The trees. My mind. The sun is reflected in the water and heating my cheeks through the frost. I hope you are listening. This outside world is very exciting, you know. It's definitely the place to be. I can't wait to introduce you to it.

Snow Baby

The snow will be gone when you come, baby.
The ice will be melting away.
A springtime bloom will be waiting for you
as soon as you come out to play.

When you open your eyes there'll be flowers
branches bloomed into hues.
The bees will be back, the petals attacked,
and the honeys will melt around you.

The white will be split when you come, baby.
The colours splintered through rain.

This blanket of snow, with its one-palette show,
will melt in a rainbow of paints.

The cold will be gone when you come, baby,
just a warm little cooling-down breeze.
The leaves on the trees will get minty and green
and the rivers run back to the seas.

The thaw will be here when you come, baby.
The animals peeping through dirt.
Daffodils trumpeting gateways to parks
as you open your ears to the earth.

The land will be soft when you sit, baby.
The grass grown through daisy-chain seats.
The sun will be bright, the heat will be light
as you lie in the shade of the trees.

The snow will be gone when you come, baby,
right now it's a blanket of pearls.
So just rest for a bit, put your feet up and sit
Till the buds break the frost and unfurl.

The freeze will be gone when you come, baby.
The glittering frost-biting tracks.

So grow strong with the Spring
and when next Winter sings
you can run out and marvel at that.

9 months pregnant – one day before due date

I panicked today and went into Mothercare to buy two baby bottles. What if I can't breastfeed? What if Dee can't get to the shops quick enough? I read that you should always have two bottles ready for the baby. The woman in the shop showed me where they were, then asked if I had a steriliser.

'No,' I said.

She said I'd need one to sterilise the bottles.

'Oh, OK,' I said. I had heard of them but hadn't got one.

She showed me different sterilising products ranging from £20 to £70 that went in the microwave.

'I don't have a microwave,' I said.

'Oh, you'll need one when you have a baby,' she laughed.

Loads of people have been telling me and Dee that – that we'll need a microwave. We'll need a microwave when we have a baby. 'You can't have a baby without a microwave,' they say. 'And a car with four doors, so it's easier to put the baby in. And a bigger flat, you'll need a bigger flat with a garden of your own, not a shared garden.'

'I don't have a microwave. Do you have any others that don't need a microwave?'

'OK,' she said, looking at me like I was an alien. 'Well, here's an electric steriliser if you don't have a microwave.'

It looked like a plastic box, but was £40 more expensive than the others and would've taken up half our kitchen.

'Do I have to have one of those?' I said.

I wasn't trying to be an annoying customer, I just didn't know a lot about all this stuff and don't have the cash to be wasting it.

She showed me two clips on the bottom of the box where the bottles could be clipped in. Then she showed me other sterilising fluid to use if I wanted to do it cold. The fluid was in bottles or sold in individual sachets like slightly larger tea bags but more plastic wrapping. Then there were sterilising tablets and quick-clean micro-steam somethings. Then she asked me if I had bottle warmers to keep the milk ready and warm for night-time feeds.

'Err, no,' I said.

I was really tired. I just wanted to get two bottles so I could feed our baby if my boobs didn't work, and I was getting more and more confused.

'Thanks,' I said, 'I'll take a look around.'

She left and I stood staring at the shelves on my own. I have no idea what I need and don't need.

An older shop assistant came over.

'I put the bottles in a saucepan and boiled them for ten minutes,' she said. 'Covered it with a plate. Or . . . ' she carried on, 'if you can breast-feed fine, nipples don't need to be sterilised and the milk will always be the right temperature. If that works, don't buy anything except breast pads and cabbages.' She walked off, smiling. I laughed and looked at the breast pumps. I figured I'd wait and see what my body could do first. I bought two bottles and nothing else.

I phoned my gran as I waddled back to the bus stop.

'Nonsense,' she said. 'You don't need a cot either, as long as you've got a big drawer or a basket or a bucket of some sort. We put my sister in the top drawer of my granddad's cupboard. And the sink makes a fine baby bath, perfect height so you don't break your back. When the war was on, the air-raid shelter in our garden also made a good sound-proof baby kennel.'

I wasn't sure if that last one was a joke or not.

My gran has lived in Glasgow all her life and she told me before that they used to threaten her little sisters and brothers with being put out in the garden when they were all huddled in the air-raid shelter, the bombings at their heaviest. My other gran got evacuated to Stirling.

Gran carried on, 'Wooden spoons and pots make good toys so don't buy any of that nonsense. And pegs. And no, love, you don't need a microwave. We did all right without that. I'm ninety-four.'

I told her she should be a personal pregnancy-shop assistant. She said she wouldn't make enough money.

Marketing Motherhood

I've stopped buying things for the baby now
Things I was told we would need
'Cos my Gran's ninety-four
and they slept in a drawer
and I feel I've been had by our shopping-land greed
That seems desperate to make money from everything it sees
They've turned death into a business deal and birth to opportunity
as a million parents just like me see the Mothercare brand
receive shopping lists for newborns handed out like birthing
        plans

Businesses marketing emotions as 'necessary buys'
as grands are spent from guilty feelings, unknown fears and
        cries

as one hundred heavy bellies walk the aisles, bulging with advice
and tags are placed on everything and unborn babies priced.

Trollies filled by worried parents,
patents push the price, declaring
products for those 'up the duff', like
If you don't buy this, you'll fuck your baby up.

Now profit margins rise each year
Collecting coins from newborn fears
Love sold in paper packets
Polkadot designer jackets
Luxury cots, Mercedes prams, nappy bags and fold-out mats
and grand-arse statements Johnson & Johnson
– Never heard such sodding nonsense
Baby oils and gels and creams
use them every day to clean,
as we hand out every ounce of cash
for creams to stop potential rash
splashing newborn skin in petrol lotion
Paraffin! Two pounds a potion!
Electric-racket baby toys
Since when did people have no voice?
Can't we read stories out ourselves?
Get a book down off the shelves?
A wooden spoon, a pan, a bell
then let them touch and see and smell.

A hundred grand for the Mothercare hug
as bankrupt parents spend for love,
told we'll mess our children up
as business rakes the profits up.

9 months pregnant

Today we both sat waiting for you but nothing happened. I'm not sure how this works now. I ate a pineapple and a vegetable tikka masala. I drank raspberry-leaf tea. Julie brought round another pineapple later on.

Everyone keeps buying me pineapples.

I went swimming. Dee took a photo of me, sent it to my dad and said it was the birthing pool. 'Is she giving birth?' my dad wrote back.

'No, but it's the due date, so we thought we'd just go to the hospital and sit in it and see what happened,' he wrote.

'Oh OK,' was the reply.

I realised none of us know much about birth, not even my dad.

'Sorry Dad, just kidding,' I text.

'Oh OK.'

Not quite the joke we'd expected. Swimming was good, though. If I was able to sleep in water right now, I would. When I'm swimming I imagine Little One inside my body swimming in my womb. A swimmer swimming in a pool inside a swimmer swimming in a pool. Cool.

1 MARCH

9 months and 1 day pregnant

7.15 p.m.

She is now overdue.

I went swimming again today. Dee's school gave us a free pass to a fancy gym. We can only use it late at night because the kids Dee teaches use it in the day.

Dee's routine these days consists of: day job at the school; night-time swimming-pool attendant for pregnant girlfriend; work at the club getting people hyped up to drum'n'bass till four a.m.; get home; refill ice tray; sleep; get up at seven a.m. to work at the school. And repeat.

Mine consists of: panicking, waddling, trying to relax, swimming, eating ice and trying to sleep.

But the pool pass is the best. The man doing lanes nearly leapt out of the pool when he saw me.

'You look ready to pop,' he said. 'When's it due?'

'Yesterday,' I replied. He got out of the pool. He actually got out of the pool.

Being in water feels so good. Getting out of the water is hard. You really are quite heavy now so if you fancy coming out any time, that would be great.

I am now more scared after seeing my naked reflection in the swimming-pool mirrors that my body is shaped like a wrong-way-round

67

triangle and the baby in my belly seems far too big for the small space between my legs.

I'm scared that I have to give birth. Birth is the biggest cause of female deaths worldwide. Thanks for the book again, Mum. I am petrified. I am shaped like a wrong-way-round triangle and I am totally fucking petrified.

In fact, I've changed my mind. I don't want to have a baby. I mean, I want a baby. I just don't want to *have* it. I want to be a man. I am scared because there is no going back now and I cannot become a man.

My mum told me to be careful last week – because my cousin lost her kidney function after birth. 'Just be careful,' she says. But how do I do that? How do I give birth carefully? I have no idea how to do this. Honestly, I am completely petrified and I live in the UK. I am also more grateful than ever that I live in the UK. That we have the NHS. We probably won't die in childbirth. But we might. And how are so many mothers and babies still dying unnecessarily in childbirth? I feel petrified and selfish. I just hope you are OK. Please let this all go OK. What can I do to make it OK? This is too much responsibility for one body to take.

'Sorry, Hollie. Sorry you have to do this. Please don't hate me,' Dee says.

'I don't hate you. I'm just scared. If I die, don't blame the baby, OK? It isn't her fault.'

'Don't say that.'

'Just promise me. Don't blame the baby. Don't hold a grudge against her.'

'OK. I won't.'

I cry.

I'm about to give birth and all I can think of is death. My mates keep asking me if I think the baby will have curly or straight hair. Blue or brown eyes? Honestly, I couldn't give a shit. Healthy. One goal. Healthy. Please. Please. Please.

Probably

I probably won't die in childbirth
I probably won't be alone
I probably won't have a ruptured aorta
I probably won't break a bone.

I probably won't be left bleeding
Or my stomach swell jumped on and bruised
I probably won't have my baby kidnapped
Or rusty knives rupture my womb.

I probably won't have to walk far
Just to be told there's no hospital space
I probably won't have infection inside me
Because I've no pennies to pay.

I probably won't have my skin ripped apart,
Fistulas spilling out faeces, for life.
I probably won't have the childbirth plight
That kills millions in labour worldwide.

8 MARCH

9 months and 8 days pregnant

4 a.m.

I woke Dee up at two a.m. as I think I'm having contractions. Whisper shakily in his ear and he leaps up out of bed quicker than I've ever seen, shouting in tired slurs, 'Fuck, cool, I'll get the car keys.'

I go to the toilet and realise I just needed a poo. Embarrassing. He goes back to sleep laughing. It's the second time I've done it this week. I tuck two pillows back under my belly and try to sleep but it's pretty impossible these days. People say, 'Get some sleep now, you won't get any when the baby's here.' Hahaha, funny. You try to sleep with a lead basketball attached to your backbone. I watch another film with a smiling couple who announce, 'We are pregnant.' I cannot stand that phrase any more. I scream at the guy on the telly: 'You are not fucking pregnant. You have no fucking idea you smug twat. And your linen shirt looks shite.' He doesn't hear me. Dee and I are having a baby. Dee is not pregnant. We are both agreed on that.

Waiting for contractions feels a bit like waiting for Christmas. It is exciting. I have no idea what contractions will actually be like. Just waiting. Awake. Waiting for an intense pain to come. Waiting for the complete unknown and a complete change of life.

'If you can still talk on the phone,' says the midwife, 'those aren't contractions. Contractions are too painful to talk through,' she laughs. Great, thanks. So I'll just wait then. Just wait for a pain so strong I can't talk. Right. Waiting. Waiting. Is that it starting? No. Be brave. Breathe. I can't sleep. I stare out of the window at the stars and cry.

Petrified.

Waiting.

Waiting.

2

SPRING
A NEW BABY

Opposite Man

Poo

Hometime

Abseil

That's Cool

Sunshine

Dream

Cheeks

Cry Like a Girl

Milk-Jug Jackers

Water Bottles

Through the Front Door

On Acid

Mermaids

Aerosmith

Stupidly Awake

Stars

Kid

Dilemma

9 months 2 weeks

24 hours in labour
  7 birthing positions
  2 parents
  1 baby – 4 hours old
  10 a.m.

First Thoughts after Birth

1. Salt-N-Pepa's 'Push It' was not as funny on the birthing CD as I had hoped.

2. I don't think I cried when the baby was born because of over-whelming motherly love. I think I cried because no one was telling me to push a bowling ball through my arse any more and I was no longer worried my ribs would break, lungs burst or face explode. Basically, labour is over and everyone is alive. I am eternally grateful and extremely lucky and will never complain about anything ever again in my life.

3. I wish someone had told me that when you have finished pushing and the baby is born, you are not done. Regardless of what the TV shows tell you, you then have to push out the placenta, which doesn't hurt but is like a huge cold jelly between your legs. You then have your legs held apart and stitches put in if you need them. That's if you have a

good birth. I am lucky. I had one stitch. I was still petrified to push out the placenta. My legs were covered in blood. No one told me my legs would be covered in blood and that the placenta would feel like cold jelly between my legs. Or that it's almost as big as the baby. The TV lies. It is all lies. I feel I have been lied to all my life. I did not look down, I was too scared to see what was there.

4. I had a good birth, I know that and I am so bloody grateful. The midwife was the greatest, most peaceful supporter I could've wished for, Dee was brilliant and everything is OK. But when the doctor came in after labour and ticked the hospital form box which was labelled 'normal/uncomplicated', I felt like punching him in the face. *Uncomplicated, you fucking think so, do you? You fucking try it then.* They should change that wording on hospital forms. At least add a 'Well done' or something.

5. I think I have joined a secret club. Why did no one tell me this stuff before? I phone up my Gran, the politest lady I have ever known. I expect her to cry with joy at the news of a new great-grandchild. She lets out a huge sigh of relief. 'Oh Hollie, I'm so glad you're OK. Fucking horrendous, isn't it?' My auntie, teacher at a local primary school, simply says, 'Shitting a watermelon?' My mum, a nurse for over thirty years and the only one I expected to ask me about the birth, just bursts out crying and cannot speak for heavy sobs, apologising as she always does when she cries. I cry too. I cry because I have no idea what to feel. I touch my stomach. It feels empty and soft and different from anything I have ever felt before. I cry because the feel of my own body is completely unknown to me and nobody warned me about that. I cry because I was just coming to terms with a pregnant body and now I need to come to terms with my body all over again. I cry because Dee is holding a baby which came out of my body. I cry because there is a baby on my chest now and she seems OK.

6. When the baby was born, she immediately crawled up the brown

magic line drawn on my belly by my skin and started sucking milk out of my nipple. Unbelievable. How did she know how to do that? She is a genius. I cry a bit more because it's all going well. I feel a bit like a cow. A bit weird. A holy Hindu cow, though. The most grateful cow on the planet.

7. I will never, ever do another poo. I will never push anything out of my body again, ever. I don't know how this will affect my digestive system but it'll just have to cope. I am told I need to do a wee but I will not. I will never do another wee or another poo ever, never, ever, never again.

8. I was forced to do a wee. After birth and the stitch and getting the baby to feed, I was taken to another room to 'relax'. I'd say 'recover', but anyway. I was given some toast and a cup of tea and told that I needed to do a wee. I was then told I couldn't leave the room to go to the main maternity ward until I did a wee. I was told to wee in the ensuite shower next to the room. They needed to know I could wee again after having a catheter up my wee hole for most of labour. I put it off for an hour. They kept coming in and asking, 'Have you done a wee yet?' They really needed the room. I cried at the thought of weeing. How can I wee now? My body is petrified to wee. Finally, I weed in the shower. I caught my reflection in the mirror, my hands shaking and all the veins in my face bright red from pushing for so long. Doing a wee has never been so scary or stinging in my life. There's no way I'll do a poo. Never. My body is broken.

9. I am not sure how to stand up holding a baby. I have only held a baby once before in my life, two weeks ago because Dee forced me to. We were visiting his cousin's newborn. Dee took the baby, passed her to me and said, 'Here's a baby, Hollie.' Then left the room. Git! I don't want to tell anyone that I don't know how to do this but I will also need to walk with the baby at some point. I'll just wait. I feel like an idiot asking how to hold my own child. I can't really walk anyway at the moment so I guess that can wait. I'm a bit scared to stand up.

10. The Russian doll is split. We came as one. We are now two separate humans and I still don't know her name. But she is happy lying on me, which is good. Maybe I'll wait till she can talk, then I'll ask her what her name is. I feel a bit weird choosing someone else's name for her.

11. I am glad I packed the really big pants. The hospital pads are like nappies. I am bleeding into a nappy and holding a baby and crying. My mum said she had a woman in hospital who brought in a thong for her change of clothes after labour. I didn't get how terrible that would be till now.

12. Dee has just phoned his mum, gran, aunts, cousins and every other mother in his family. Firstly to tell them he has a healthy baby. Secondly to congratulate them all for giving birth. 'Seriously,' I hear him say. 'Well done, Grandma. Seven, though?' He is in shock. I am too. His new-found respect for mothers is immense. Mine too. I hear him congratulating every one he has ever known over the telephone. 'Thanks, Mum. No really, thanks, Mum.'

'Well done, Hollie,' he says. He looks at me, holding the baby against his chest. 'We've got a baby.' And he cries. And I cry again, too. I think I am crying out of love now. But I am not sure. I am really tired. The baby is the only person not crying. The bravest one of us all.

Opposite Man

He's the opposite of what the article said.
It said:
'Reconsider dad's place by the hospital bed.'
Nemesis of generations gone
of men spouting the same old song
of women's Instinct, maternal minds.
Through male and macho crap you shine

Dripping energy onto my tongue
in bottled drinks and calming songs
As shivers took my body hold
and vessels burst in birthing groans

You grabbed her
You cleaned her first
You cut the cord
You saw the worst or as you seem to say
The best
A man could ever see.

Granddad didn't dare.
Told to sit outside with concerned stares
Puffing smoke to passing ticks
No concept of what women did.
You stand opposite to history
The sight, how like some crowned glory,
While other men brush off and say that
'gory birth' is not their taste.
I feel the pain is soothed by praise
you brag about my strength today
The things I really wanna shout
but am told a 'lady' won't let out.

As women undermine themselves,
Underplay the pain they felt,
We need more men like you
To tell the tale of what we all go through

You're the opposite of what the article said,
That 'men shouldn't be at the hospital bed'

'Cos you calmed me, laughed, through a roomful of pain
And now you shout out the strengths that I'm not meant to
     claim

13. But there's another guy who I hear talking. 'I don't do nappies,' he says, in front of his partner. They have two kids. He just doesn't do nappies. Doesn't like it. Nah. I cannot get this. It didn't bother me so much before – hearing men say this. I've heard it a lot before. But now, after all this, after actually knowing what it is like to be pregnant and give birth, I imagine pouring the nappy contents over his head. Immature I know, but.

Poo

'I don't do nappies,' spouts from this man's mouth
And I'm awake when I should sleep 'cos the fire won't go out.
Flames burn in my belly, angry tears on cheek
At the sexist attitude that baby-care can reek.
He just 'doesn't do nappies', says
He just 'doesn't like the poo'
As if women, wives or mothers naturally fucking do.
And after all the worry that the baby mother went through
Crying, rocks and cuddles are as much as he will do.
She carries it for nine months in morning sickness reigns
Body morphs as baby grows and back groans intense pains
Fearing any move she makes might affect the child inside her
No alcohol, no drugs at all, constant worries grind her.
Then labour pain, sometimes for days
And childbirth, there's no words to say
The movie horror beauty gaze of how it feels for her that day
As nature has its way and well OK I just won't go that way.

But let's just say, though others may
I won't forget the strain today.
Then they take the kid back home
Her belly sags and boobs explode
A milk machine life-giving throne
Breasts cramp each time the baby groans
Nipples leak and stitches stick
Discomfort like no one can give
And after this, on top of it
She wakes each three hours to feed the kid.
And after all that women do
He says, 'Oh no, I don't like poo.'
If you were mine, here's what I'd do.
Forget the kid.
I'll poo on you.

I need to sleep.
    This baby is magic.

4 p.m.

'You can go home now,' the nurse smiled.

I didn't want to go home. I have no idea what I'm doing. But the ward was boiling hot and sitting with a baby, listening to women in the labour ward screaming screams louder than I have ever heard in my life, was a bit like being in the middle of a new interactive horror film. For some reason the screams were worse to hear after I had given birth. I guess I could picture it more. I don't know why I didn't scream much. I guess just because in general I don't really shout or scream. Never have. I didn't swear or lash out at Dee. I think he was a bit disappointed. I didn't break his hand or tell him I hated him, another popular movie scene. I just sat and pretended I was a Buddha and secretly pressed my palm on my clit to distract the nerves from the pain in the rest of my body. A friend told me to do that, but it's an unspoken thing, I realise. Annoying that, seeing as it's the female spot with the most number of nerve endings and therefore the best spot on your body which could in any way take pressure off the intensity of the labour pains. Like a rush of paracetamol. But in prudish Britain people would imagine you're trying to finger yourself into labour and possibly call you a dirty, sex-obsessed, weirdo slut mother. Finger on your own clit – number one sin worldwide – nice.

Anyway, it was horrible going home. Nine hours after a child came out of a nine-month stint inside my body. Me. With no experience of babies. Or breastfeeding. Or bathing. Or anything. I walked really slowly out of the ward and burst into tears. I thought my ribcage was missing. I panicked. I started feeling about for my ribs. I couldn't find them. I started breathing too quickly.

'Are you OK, Hollie?' Dee said.

'I have no idea, I don't know what's normal to feel right now. My body is battered. I just don't know what's OK and what's not.'

My whole body's insides have shifted to make space for a baby who is currently being carried by her dad, leaving a baby-sized gap inside my body as my organs slowly shift back into place. I guess I imagined it'd all happen straight away, pop-up-tent style, which is stupid, I know. My ribcage feels like it's too high and I can't breathe. I tried to find my ribs again and they felt like they were round my neck. It scared me. I didn't want to go home. We went back into the ward and asked the receptionist again.

'Well you can wait, but a doctor could be half an hour, or eight hours,' she said. I smiled and walked out of hospital trying to hide the tears. I just wanted someone there to understand that I was petrified and to give a shit about it. I wanted the nice midwife back. Dee held my hand and we left.

Hometime

But it is good to be home.
It is good to be home with our new flatmate.
So what happens now?
We stare at a baby sleeping on a blanket on our bed.
So what happens now?
Nothing, she carries on sleeping.
We sit in silence, drinking tea, staring at a small person
    sleeping.
Waiting. But not for pain this time. It's much nicer now.
Waiting.
Waiting.
She carries on sleeping.
I cannot believe there was actually a baby inside me. A real one.

14 MARCH

1 day old

Then visitors flock like flies. All eyes on the baby and me.

I can't wee properly and when I do I have to rinse with water in the shower because you're not allowed to use toilet paper for a while afterwards in case of infection. But no one told me about that. Everyone says how well I look and I feel a bit sorry for Dee. Everyone makes their own tea. Someone even says I look thinner, which I find a bit strange. I have muslin cloths that we bought for the baby shoved down my pants because the hospital pads don't really do the job and no one told me that I would be bleeding so I didn't have time to shop. No one told me I would be bleeding, as if I would just guess. But I didn't guess.

And I am bleeding.

My breasts are leaking.

I am feeding.

I am crying.

I am knackered.

The day is full of guests.

Then everything stops.

Everyone leaves.

And it's just him and me and the baby.

And he needs to sleep so we're not *both* zombies and I don't want to go to bed because it feels like a joke lying in a bed when you are blatantly not going to sleep.

So I sit on the settee
  And he kisses our heads and leaves.
  And from two a.m. to six a.m., baby, it's just you and me.

Abseil

As you abseil down my chest like a miniature rock climber
Hands grip tightly, push off from my shoulder-blade cliffs
You career from left to right, mind focused, eyes open
No waterproofs or harness, just a purple Babygro
You stop, grunting for assistance, I see panic setting in
Until quick fingers grope the spot
and you fling your head across the sky
to your chosen side
and land
Lips clamped and drink
Then you fall asleep from the exertion
My hungry, extreme-sports baby
abseil down me
any time.

That's Cool

You like to kick at five a.m., that's cool, I like to write
You like to rock at three a.m., that's cool, I like the night
You like to gaze out windowpanes, that's cool, I like the light
You like to lie upon my chest, that's cool, I like the sight.

2 p.m.

Today the milk 'came in'. I never quite understood what that meant. What it means is that my boobs felt like they were about to explode. Hard, solid as a rock, sore and growing like the water balloons that Caroline, Jodie and me just kept filling as kids before we climbed onto the top of Sally's shed and threw them down on our older siblings. Panicking, I asked my dad to get a breast pump, genuinely worried they wouldn't stop filling up. He was too embarrassed. My breasts are exploding milk, between my legs is bleeding continuously and the baby is crying. And the room is full of visitors. But I don't really want to chat. I want to put on my big pants and go to sleep. I really want to go to sleep. My mum says my boobs won't explode and pumping milk will just make them produce more 'cos they're so goddamn clever. When the baby drinks it feels like she's slowly releasing air from an over-pumped monster truck tyre. She's the only one that can do it. Drink, please, drink!

I go for a wee and shower off and then for some reason I feel for the stitch inside. Or maybe I'm just curious to see what my body feels like down there. I go for it. It feels completely different. I think I feel a stitch, but I'm not sure. Something wiry in between a more jelly-like texture than I've ever known before. I panic again and stop. I don't recognise my own body. It looks different and it feels different. I can't stop thinking about how, just when I was getting used to being pregnant, my body has completely changed and I have to get used to it all over again. So when I'm used to it again, what will happen then? If I ever do.

Every time someone tells me how well I look, I want to cry. I want to tell them how weird it is; how my skin is now empty; how I've never seen my body like this; or any body like this, ever; how I'm finding that hard to deal with because nothing around me tells me this is a good look. I want to tell them not to talk about how I look right now. Every time someone tells me how lovely the baby is, I feel guilty and upset and confused. Because she is lovely, she is healthy and happy and that

87

should be my main thought. And it is one of my thoughts. But I also feel scared and upset and sort of trapped and worried and tired. I do feel happy too. I do feel well. It's just every time someone else tells me that, I feel terrible for having any other thoughts. I can't wait to get to know this little person properly. And to get to know my body again, too.

Last night she didn't seem to be getting any milk. As it was one a.m. and I had nothing better to do, I sat and watched. She spent at least half an hour fiddling with my nipple. She blew on it, tweaked it until she felt the milk come into it, then she patted it with her hand to make it hard enough to use as a teat. I did nothing, I sat and watched like an out-of-body experience. It took a while, it took nearly an hour, but when the milk was in and the teat done, she drank and it worked. I did nothing, she did it all. She is a bloody genius. I am a vessel. I am slightly weirded out by this. Fascinated too. She is totally cool with it, which is the most important thing. I need to learn from her. It annoys me that I find this feeding stuff weird when it is so brilliant.

15 MARCH

3 days old

Dee had a gig last night. He said he didn't have to go but I insisted. Before Little One was born we spoke a lot about carrying on working, not giving up gigs. Working day jobs and night jobs and having a baby is a bit odd. His set was two a.m. until four a.m. The entire time he was gone I didn't move. I sat up in bed with my arms in a cradle trying not to wake her and staring at her face. I sat through extreme pins and needles, through being desperate for the toilet, because I am so scared to break this tiny, tiny person. Get back in my body please. No, don't. When I think about labour, it's like having nightmare flashbacks. I know that sounds bad, but that's what it's like for me. I still cannot believe what labour was like.

Anyway, after a two-hour stint standing on stage emceeing at another drum'n'bass rave, Dee came back. 'Everything OK?' he said, and took her from me. 'Yep,' I said, trying not to show that I could hardly move my legs and arms from the position they'd been fixed in for two hours. Dee and Little One seem to know how to do everything somehow. He's so good with babies. I don't know how to do anything.

One of my friends said she didn't want to leave her baby with his dad for a few hours because he wouldn't know what to do. But neither do I. I have no sodding idea what to do right now. And neither will my friend's partner if he's never allowed to look after his baby. I don't know why we assume it's different for guys. It's so much more down to how much experience you have with babies. Not what gender you are.

Soon I will learn how to put you down without waking you up. And how to hold you properly. And how to bath you. And how to be a parent. And how not to be so scared to move. You're pretty good at being a baby though. Well done.

It is pretty wonderful, this life cycle. I always found it interesting, how food is made and seeds grow and sunshine and rain become nutrition and we eat and poo and seeds grow and so on. But now my body is taking that and making a whole new product and there is another little human being joining in my loop of life. I can't get my head round it all. This brilliant earth. My brilliant digestive system.

Sunshine

Baby, I can't tell you what a pleasure it is to feed you
Feet up in a dim-lit room, nothing but life between us
Milky silent gulping, face a blissful rest
Tiny fingers tapping on the spaces by my chest
Bellies beat together, slowly in and out
Heartbeats storm through tiny chest, tinted lips and
      mouth
As I sit and wait, I gaze again at our cherry blossom tree
As light to leaf to the air we breathe, now that system flows
      through me
And as I gaze upon your face, pressed upon me
I see the cycle,
our food recycled,
as you gulp down sunshine energy.

3.40 a.m.

Dream

When you laugh in your sleep, I smile in my wake
Knowing some dream has floated your way

When you laugh wide awake I wanna smile till I cry
Peace in your signal that something is right.

3.44 a.m.

Cheeks

When I watch them both sleep
I wanna bite both their cheeks
I mean, his and hers.
I mean, face and bum.

4.15 a.m.

I watch her crying and I cry because she won't stop crying. I hope she'll stop. Then she stops and falls asleep and laughs. I think it's incredible that before we can talk or walk or run, we cry and laugh and smile. Crying at birth is a sign of life. It was all I hoped she would do when she was born. So why do we see it as weak when we're older? I cry a bit more. Tired tears and happy tears and 'What the fuck is going on?' tears. It feels good to cry – important, almost.

A woman in town told her little boy to stop crying the other day. 'You're not a little girl,' she said. I think that's a shame. It must be hard for little boys. And big ones too, actually. I think next time I'm dissed by a guy about why the hell I'm crying, I'll just ask him why the hell he's *not*. 'What's the matter with you? Why aren't you crying? Why don't you ever cry?'

It is such a dangerous part of our culture, the fear of letting liquid loose from our eyes.

Cry Like a Girl

I drive like a girl and I cry like a girl
Young men's suicide rates are too high in this world
I cry like a girl, I won't bottle it in.
I cry like a girl.
That's a good thing.

I cry like a girl and I drive like a girl
Young men's motoring deaths are too high in this world
I drive like a girl, I don't pose, speed or spin.
I drive like a girl.
That's a good thing.

So I'll keep crying it out.

5 days old

This is all so odd. Funny and odd. Little One came off my nipple before she'd finished yesterday and a stream of milk shot into her face and then across the room. In the shower, I put up my arms and both boobs shot milk out in sharp, dagger-like lines like the Austin Powers movie. Dee's finding it hilarious. I find it funny sometimes, but also really strange. Other times it makes me feel a bit sick if I'm honest, a bit too much like a cow. Sometimes I'm like 'Come and look at this!' Other times it's more 'Stop looking at me.' But I am really blessed I can do it. Despite the cramps and the wet, smelly T-shirts and milk stains and sore boobs, there haven't been any problems. I know I'm lucky.

She is a monster, she growls at my boob for milk, drinks, then lies back completely drunk. Dee calls her 'the milk-jug jacker'. I imagine her like a drunk robber sat in a milk bar. I write another poem for her. Maybe one day she'll read it. I nick his title. He won't mind. I gave birth to his child, for God's sake. She is sleeping and I wonder if she dreams. Do babies dream? I think if she does, this might be how it goes:

Milk-Jug Jackers

Baby you look tired, where have you been?
My baby girl smiles gummy and looks up at me.

She says, 'Mummy every morning between midnight and three
We go milk-jug-jacking all my babies and me.
We meet in secret on the green just outside the flats
The babies, bunnies, birds and the cats
We sit on bunnies' backs, galloping, and follow the birds
The cats' eyes light the path of the outside world.
To the big park lakes is where we run
Where, waiting by the piers, are our friendly swans.
We jump off bunnies' backs to the white swans' wings
Sit amongst the feathers where we whisper and sing:
"We are the milk-jug jackers and we're coming your way
Ladies better watch out, put your nipples away
We've got our crowbars at the ready to snap off your straps
Happy slapper milk-jug jackers, hope you're ready for that."
With our animal friends and our bunny-rabbit cars
We sit, snapping bras, in our milk-jug bars
Till our potbellies are full of white baby rum
Then the swans fly us home for our feed time with mum
Sipping on your nipple I giggle in delight
'Cos you don't know I've been drinking milk in all the night.
Sipping on your nipple I giggle in delight
'Cos you don't know I've been milk-jug-jacking all of the night.'

19 MARCH

1 week old

4.15 a.m.

This week has been good, I think. Though I still have no idea what I am doing. Dee has shown me how to change nappies and bath a baby. He was the older cousin, I was the youngest. He makes it look so easy. I have slept, roughly, an hour a night. How do people do this on their own? I don't get it. More funding for single parents. Sleep deprivation is used to torture people, and some parents are on their own, getting just one hour's sleep a night with no help. I can't imagine what that's like. Hard, very hard, and way underestimated. Frowned upon, even.

Dee says his new role is filling up water bottles. Breastfeeding makes me so thirsty. I haven't quite worked out how to move when she sleeps, which is causing a few issues at night-time. I get pins and needles a lot. Last night was the most successful one yet. I didn't cry as much as the others.

Water Bottles

On the first night:
He put a cup of water on the table next to us
before he went to bed
he kissed our heads

and when he woke again
we were sitting on the other sofa
by the window, I was
staring at the cup of water
that was just slightly too far.
At three a.m. I moved
to look out at the stars
'cos she was crying
and after an hour of trying
she fell asleep at last
I took the chance to sit down
and sat down in the wrong place
and I'm so thirsty now I ache
and I didn't want to wake her
and she cried each time I tried to move
and I didn't know what to do
and I haven't been to sleep yet
and my mouth is really dry
and I really want to cry
and then I cried.
I'm not very good at this, am I?

On the second night:
He put one cup of water on the table
and one across the room
another on the desk
and a last one in the bathroom
'Just in case,' he laughed
and then
he went to bed again
and I fed her
and she fell asleep

and I reached out and found a glass of water right there next to
    me
I breathe out and smile
and I put it to my lips
as tiny moves of tiny feet kick
the icy drink all over me.
My pyjamas soaked, but baby dry,
I cried
that night
sitting quiet from three a.m. till daylight
wet trousers, wet crotch,
not knowing what to do
he came inside at six a.m.
with toast and jam and fruit
'Why didn't you wake me?'
'I do not know,' I said.
With damp cold on my thigh and legs
he took the Little One aside
I changed my clothes and lay in bed
and cried.
I'm not very good at this, am I?

On the third night:
He put the water into bottles
on every surface of the room
and bottles do not leak
because lids can be screwed on
and after he had gone to bed
and kissed our heads
and she was fed,
staring at her tiny face
I placed her hand in mine

and I cried again.
'I'm not good at this,' I whispered
and I'm sure she winked a bit
I look into her eyes
and I cry.

I cry because my crotch is dry
I cry 'cos I am so damn tired
I cry because she smiled
I cry 'cos I can reach a drink
I cry because her lips look a little bit like his
and I can sit and see her properly at last.

24 MARCH

12 days old

4 a.m.

I can't stop thinking about two things:

1. The Bounty saleswoman who was allowed into our hospital ward straight after birth. I've been thinking about it since we came back, and more and more I'm angry about it. We didn't realise she was a saleswoman. We thought she was from the NHS. But I've looked in the 'hospital pack' now and feel stupid. She was definitely just a businesswoman sales representative.

2. The fact that we have already got vouchers and leaflets related to babies coming through our flat's front door. Who gave out our address to companies already?

Through the Front Door

My mum couldn't come to the hospital
because only one guest was allowed
My dad couldn't visit and friends couldn't pass by
to see the new mum and dad proud
and that's fine, I don't mind, until two hours past labour
our hospital door was pushed open
and a sales representative from Bounty or something

strolled in with a bag full of potions.
Sales pitches and leaflets and pamper club vouchers
and samples of Johnson's baby shampoos
Too stunned after labour, in my head I couldn't savour
'And who in hell's name are you?'
And now at home the post is piled high with adverts
and coupons off Pampers' new pamphlets
and discount-code vouchers from Asda
and Boots
and Johnson & Johnson
and I thought after pondering
How the hell did these companies get to our door so fast?
And who passes addresses of fresh-fragile parents
to strangers from businesses and brands?
'Cos isn't it dangerous to let people know
every name and door number of every new home
where parents lie sleeping or a parent alone
with a new baby crying and insides that groan?
Like an invite to burglars or robbers or thieves:
In this house is a person who can't up and leave
or stand up or fight
and had no sleep last night
so come on inside if you're up for the ride!
I didn't know it's legal
I think it should change
to let sales people pester new parents' brains
to give companies our addresses and names
when we have a new baby at home.
It's insane
Surely that law should be changed?

24 MARCH

12 days old

We got a letter through the post today telling us we have to name our baby before the deadline. I wonder what happens if you miss it? The baby is never allowed a name? They pick a name at random?

13 days old

2 p.m.

I have started a feeding diary to remind me if it's night-time or day-time or feeding time or sleep time or poo time. It feels a bit like being on acid, this. Minus the party first. Minus the music. Eat. Sleep. Poo. Repeat. Eat. Sleep. Poo. Repeat.

Three a.m. left boob – sleep. Four-fifteen a.m. poo – wee – change. Five a.m. right boob – sleep. Poo. Sleep. Right boob. Left boob. Left boob again. Left. Right. Left. Left. Right.

I've noticed I'm dreaming a lot, but they never finish. My dreams don't get to finish any more. Dream. Scream. Wake. Right, left, right, left.

4.55 a.m.

On Acid

I'm living a life of half-dreams
Sleep interrupted in breastmilk streams
Adventures broken in two a.m. screams
Eyes open and closing like counting machines
Between two-hour shifts where I swap with me

I'm living a life of half-dreams
Cellophane flowers and tangerine trees
Rowing down milk rivers through breast-hill valleys
To nipple-cream islands in cold cups of tea

I'm living a life of half-dreams
Comatose arms rock automatically
Tiny lips to my breast my mind tries to see
If she's just fed and I've fallen or if she's waiting to feed
If she's just fed or she's hungry or if I'm already asleep

I'm living a life of half-dreams
Asleep with ears open, checking she breathes
Staring at ceilings to birds' melodies
Singing in day as I drift back to sleep

I'm living a life of half-dreams
Stories stolen by waking bellies
Body jolts upright with every night scream
Eye bags, arm muscles, breasts are heavy

I'm ready in every half-dream
Waking to two big eyes staring at me
With a fist stuffed in mouth to ease the need
As she waits for my waking with impatient greed

I was lying in bed. Wake up. Breastfeed.
I was dreaming I slept. Wake up. Breastfeed.
I was dreaming we kissed. Wake up. Breastfeed.
I was dreaming your lips. Wake up. Breastfeed.
I was sleeping. She wept. Wake up. Breastfeed.
I was awake as she slept. Wake up. Breastfeed.

I fell asleep as she fed. Wake up. Breastfeed.
I woke up as you said. Wake up. Breastfeed.
She finished. She smiled. Our eyes met.
Wake up. Breastfeed. It's blessed.

26 MARCH

Nearly 2 weeks old

Dee goes back to his day job this week. Two weeks' paternity leave is over, the school kids are waiting for him and I am petrified again. I am hiding it and smiling but I'm really fucking scared. I feel like I just about know how to hold a baby now. Feeding is fine. Sleep is not. I am really scared of being on my own with her all day. Especially when I'm so tired. What if something goes wrong? What if she's sick or ill? How will I eat? How will I get to the loo? How will I wash the blood or change my pads? What if she vomits in the shops? What if? What if? I want Dee to stay home with me some more. Everyone says 'You'll be fine', but I know it'll be hard and the pressure of being the sole person responsible for a tiny baby is building up. I'm really nervous about Dee going back to work. About doing this on my own. Especially leaving the flat by myself. And I have to leave the flat because if I stay in, she cries and I start to get cabin fever. Stay-at-home parent, my arse. It's the worst phrase I've ever heard to describe this. It seriously needs to be changed because it gives the wrong message out to everyone. No one with a baby is ever at home. Pushing-a-pram-like-a-zombie-round-the-streets-stressing-continually-about-what-the-matter-is parent might be a better description

27 MARCH

2 weeks old

9 p.m.

I was reading a newspaper article with Little One lying on my legs today. Sixty-one people died off the coast of Tripoli, including two babies. Fleeing for their lives, they drifted at sea for two weeks, dying of thirst, and even though their boat had been located by the authorities, no one came to help them. 'African refugees' they are called in the newspaper. So people then, yeah? They are people. And babies. Survivors told how helicopters and boats all came towards them as they sat on a boat at sea, saw them as they signalled the dead bodies and their need for water. The helicopter crews didn't help, but left them for dead. NATO was supposedly controlling this and did nothing, even when an emergency alarm was called by the Italian island of Lampedusa. I just cannot get my head around this world. World leaders, Gadaffi, NATO, playing with people's lives.

So people, including two babies, same flesh and blood as any baby, lie at the bottom of the sea, because a group of old fucking political leaders are too wrapped up in their own greed and goddamn egos. Two babies floated to the bottom of the sea this month, when they could've been easily saved. People dead on boats with rescue helicopters miles away who fully understood their situation. Who do you think you are? And all we do is sit and watch shite game shows and cooking programmes and do crossword puzzles while it goes on. And worry about how to decorate the nursery, as if our babies give a damn about the choice of carry-mat their shitty bums are changed on or the patterns on their walls. I feel a bit sick today. I wonder what I could have done in the time it took me to choose her playmat. I wonder what playmat those babies had before they were forced onto an inflatable boat and out to sea, to flee their country. I wonder what colour their blankets were. I wonder what their names were. I hold her as tight as possible. I don't know if I'll ever be able to let go.

Mermaids

I hope they find you, baby
On playmat ocean floors
I hope they make you seaweed sheets and wrap you warm on
    sandy reefs
I hope the corals sway for you, your oyster rattles clutched in
    hands
Pearls shake with open-eyed amazement watching seahorse
    bubble bands
I hope the mermaids sing for you and curve the waves to lull
    your sleep
I hope your tears are wiped by mother octopuses' eight great feet
I hope you land so softly, babies, float onto the ocean's floor
And hope that we learn up above to welcome people to our
    shores
To help them out of fleeing boats
and let them live upon safe lands

Too late for you.
I pray you both sank safely into mermaids' hands.

Aerosmith

And now I feel like I know why love songs are written
And I finally know what I really believe in

What I would die for
Lose spirit and life for
Stand in front of gunfire
and firing lines for

And I don't mean to be too loud or sound like a bore but
I feel like I understand my meaning of life more now.

My eyes are glued to you, baby, I think they're stuck for good. I can't let you out of my sight. I finally get that Aerosmith song. I think it was about Liv, not his lover. It was about his daughter, for sure. 'I don't wanna close my eyes, I don't wanna fall asleep 'cos I miss you babe and I don't wanna miss a thing.' In my head, I sound just like Steven Tyler singing it ... 'I don't wanna faaaaaaaaaalllllllllll asleeeeeeepp. Dah dah Dahhhhh.' It reminds me of school discos. Let's slow-dance.

Stupidly Awake

When I've had a week of twelve a.m. three a.m. five a.m. wakes
A new mum awake in a zombie-like state
When you do go to sleep
and I need to sleep too
I spend another three hours just staring at you.

When I've had a week of one a.m. three a.m. six a.m. wakes
and my eyelids spend days in a half-closed/shut state
When you do fall asleep
and I need to sleep too
I can't help staying up just to gaze down at you.

When I've had a week of twelve a.m. two a.m. four a.m. wakes
and all my energy's used just to keep me awake
When you do get to sleep
and I must go to bed
I spend another two hours just stroking your head.

1 month old

4 p.m.

What am I doing to myself? Sleep, Hollie, sleep. It's just not that easy. I'm not a robot. I feel like screaming this out to everyone I know. I cannot sleep on demand, even when I am more tired than I thought was humanly possible.

My mum took Little One around the park for an hour yesterday, 'So you can get some sleep, Hollie.' When she came back I'd made a lasagne for our lunch. She shouted at me. I felt like I was fifteen again. My mum never shouts.

So I've started lying. Dee took Little One out last week. 'So you can sleep, Hollie.' I couldn't sleep. He came back and first thing he said was 'Did you get some sleep?'

What I actually did was lie on the sofa, close my eyes, realise I couldn't sleep, then get up and try on a dress. Put on Ms Dynamite's second album – which in some ways I like more than the award win-ning first one, reminds me a lot of Tanya Stephens – and crash out in the middle of the floor singing along to the first three tracks. I switched it off, made a cup of tea and drank it while it was hot, listening to the beautiful silence of the flat and breathing in the steam like it was fairy dust. I ran back to the bedroom, changed back into my tracksuit and as I heard Dee walk in through the door I lay down and pulled the cover over me, trying to be as quiet as I could.

'Did you sleep, Hollie?'

'Yes I did, thanks,' I said, trying to sound yawny.

I lied. Because I appreciate him so much and about ninety per cent of the time, I do sleep, or at least close my eyes and rest. I am so grateful to him, even if I'm slightly bored with thanking Dee and others all the time for letting me do things that were just normal life before. Thank you for letting me go to the loo on my own; thank you for letting me try to go to sleep for twenty minutes; to have a shower by myself. But I do appreciate it a lot, and I want them to know that and to feel helpful, because they are. I couldn't do this alone, no way. It's just that I don't like being told what to do with my one hour alone each week. I don't like being ordered to sleep. I am an adult. I am a mum. And people keep telling me what to do with the smidgen of time I have to myself.

'So you can sleep, Hollie.'

'So you can sleep, Hollie.'

'So you can sleep, Hollie.'

'Sleep now, Hollie. Right now, Hollie. If you don't, then don't complain about being tired because you had your chance of an hour's catch-up.'

I can feel them thinking that everytime they take Little One and I don't sleep. But an hour's nap each day won't make up for six months of five a.m. morning sickness, three months of heavy-belly sleeping troubles, a twenty-hours-awake labour process and one hour's sleep a night since then. But it is definitely better than none.

So this time I spent an hour listening to the radio and cooking lasagne while my mum walked Little One round the park.

'Why did you make a flaming lasagne?' she shouted. 'You had an hour to sleep!'

Because I couldn't fucking sleep, OK? I didn't say it like that. I love my mum.

Because I couldn't, I said. Because I miss cooking, I said. Because I miss doing things other than feeding and changing fucking nappies and trying to sleep and being worried about whether I'm doing it all wrong. I know how to cook a lasagne. Because I miss having a little time by myself to do something that adults do. And it felt so good to have the flat to myself and cook a meal for my mum.

She gives me a hug.

'Sorry, love, it's just because I remember being so tired all the time because my lot weren't close. I just don't want you to be so exhausted.'

'Thanks, Mum. Do you want some lasagne?'

Last night Dee said, 'I'm just popping to Pete's house,' and I replied, 'I hate you.'

I really miss being able to say 'I'm just popping out.' He laughed. I laughed.

'I don't hate you really,'

'Yes, you do,' he said.

'I don't! Yeah I do, sorry. Only when you say "I'm just popping out." Or when you don't have to ask to go to the loo. Or to have a shower. Or to breathe by yourself for a second.'

It's really frustrating having to ask permission to do everything.

'Excuse me, could you hold the baby so I could please go and do a poo and wipe my arse? Oh thank you so much.'

But I can't complain. Dee holds Little One every minute he gets a chance. Not when he's asked, just when he's there. Because he wants to hold his baby. He takes her out. Puts her to bed. Bathes her. Changes her nappies. I see loads of mums who have to ask their partners to do anything.

'Would you mind bathing her tonight?'

'Would it be OK if you took her for a walk?'

'Could you please hold your *own child* just this once so I can eat my sodding dinner – which is already cold 'cos you've eaten yours first?'

Not even a question of getting time on their own to just chill. No chance. I think this is where hatred starts between a lot of couples. Deep-seated resentment. If I couldn't tell Dee I hate him sometimes, I don't think we'd work. I wouldn't cope. I think I'd turn violent.

So Dee pops out to see his mates. I watch him leave enviously. Then Little One smiles at me. I smile back, feeling guilty but in love.

10 p.m.

Stars

I still get excited staring at stars
Eyes in awe, calm, baby bundle now in arms
Through the curtain gap, I dream away
fascination takes away the pain that
it's not day
and I'm awake
and shouldn't be
and need to sleep.

I still get excited staring at stars
Especially the ones that sail in fast
with two red lights on plane-tip wings
I daydream I'm up there, strapped in
sipping tea from plastic cups
engine whirrs to keep me up
rather than my baby's grunts
and heavy breaths
and snoring.

I see the aisle lights bright as day
off to some much warmer place

I wonder who is up there now
peering down on mapped-out towns

Then I look down and see your face
and I'm happy just to gaze.

Kid

Since I've had a kid I feel like one again
desperate for a steering hand
my mother's help – extra hugs
reassurance that I'm doing great
whilst not knowing what the fuck I'm doing.

I'm like a learning, yearning kid again
since I had a kid.

1½ months old

23.32 p.m.

Dilemma

When she finally sleeps, I mean *finally* sleeps
Like that eyes rolled back, lips apart deep kinda sleep
No peeks, eyes relaxed, closed no leaks thick kinda sleep
Heavy breaths keep to meeting heartbeats kinda sleep
When she finally sleeps, I mean finally sleeps
And our bed sheets haven't been seen for days kinda sleep,
And it seems we've got three full hours before her next feed
And we sneak into bed and our legs want to weep,
Finally, lying down, her father and me –
The dilemma appears like a newborn, brutally.

'Cos she finally sleeps, we can finally be
Skin to skin, cuddled under covers in glee
Our giggling eyelids smile heavily
As we shoosh at each sound that might wake the baby
One kiss on your cheek to tell you goodnight
One kiss on your lips and a hand to your thighs

As your head wants to dream and there isn't much time
But the warmth of the back of your body on mine
Three hours turn to two to tease me awake
And your breath feels so good on my aching neck nape
But each kiss that I give is one more minute awake
And I haven't slept well for at least twenty days
If I carry the play on, keep touching your face,
We won't get the sleep our minds desperately crave
Fulfilling a space, my skin endings ache.
But I panic each second we're still both awake
I want to keep touching but I desperately don't
I want the hours to lengthen but they desperately won't
As I drift back and forth from your body to lone
And the bed drifts from sensual to sleep-giving throne
Moaning, both body and mind,
At the choice between sanity and feeling your sighs
The dilemma awakens each wonderful time
She finally sleeps
And your body's with mine.

20 MAY

2 months old

In the Back Room

I did my first poetry gig today after having Little One. In Peterborough. I booked it before Little One was born as I thought it'd be fine. And it was. I felt really chuffed. Mum came and like an underpaid angel just hung around and held Little One all day. I gave a feed before I went in. I had to judge thirty young poets, aged ten upwards, and it was lovely. It was lovely doing something different. After watching all the young people (with no crying from Little One), there was a break before we went into the back room to decide the winners. I took her for a feed and went into the corner of the back room, facing the window, my back facing the other three judges who sat chatting round the table. I fed her in the ten-minute break. Perfect timing. After she was fed, Mum took her again and I joined the other judges. Great poets, Mark Grist, Tim Clare, MC Mixy. All male, young poets. All brilliant.

Then after the day was done, prizes awarded, poems heard, the organiser of the whole thing, the man who had asked me specifically to do the gig when I was heavily pregnant, said: 'I don't think you should've done this if you couldn't cope, Hollie. I don't think it was very professional, what you did.'

Today was the first day I have felt properly shit about motherhood in this way. I was feeding a baby in the corner of a back room, my face to the wall like a dunce-cap kid. That was my choice, possibly a stupid one. And for feeding my baby, perfectly timed in between poetry sets, for doing a fifteen-minute set with no problems, I'm told I'm 'not professional'. The only female judge out of a panel of four in his competition. The only female performer, and he tells me that. I did everything the others did, I performed, I judged, I watched, I scored. Baby was an angel, she didn't cry once for me and no one even saw her. She fed when she was told to. Mum took a day off from her own job to drive three-and-a-half hours to help me do this. But I'm not fucking professional. We're not fucking professional.

Breathe in, Hollie. Breathe in. To be honest, I thought Mum was going to deck him before I did.

Breathe in. It's just him. He's just a knob. The other guys didn't bat an eyelid.

21 MAY

2 months old

This month is kind of rolling into one long daydream, broken up every so often with Dee's or my mum coming to help, me and Dee going out, and baby group. I am so thankful for the local baby group – a group of mainly seventy-year-old women (there is one seventy-year-old man too) who, three times a week, open up their church hall for tired parents to have a rest and a hot cup of tea and a biscuit while their babies roll about and play. Despite the initial awkwardness of sitting with people I don't know at all and the worry that because it's in a church I might not be as welcome, it really is heaven. I look forward to the tea all morning before the group starts. It is the best tea and biscuit I've ever had in my life. Ever. And it is good to see that the other parents seem to be just as stumbling as me. I am so thankful for my mum's help, for Dee's mum and for all those making the tea and biscuits at baby group. Just sorry none of them are getting paid. Seems to be an awful lot of women around me not getting paid for any of this work.

So the breaks are great. But the days and nights are getting pretty repetitive:

I feed her and she sleeps and I sleep and she wakes and I wake and I feed her and she wakes and he helps and he holds her so I sleep and she sleeps and I feed her and we go out and we come back and the tea's cold and I feel crap and I feel great and I feel calm and I wonder about my life this far and I cry and I weep and I breathe in and I breathe out and baby group is like a heaven where the tea is always hot and I sob and I stop and I feed her and she sleeps and I sleep and I don't sleep and I cry if she sleeps and I smile and I scream and I laugh and she laughs and I cry and she sleeps and days and nights blur into one and we walk and she sleeps and I stop and she wakes and he holds her and he goes out and we fight a bit and he laughs a bit and he holds her so I sleep and I don't sleep and I cry and we laugh and she laughs and we smile because she's all right with us, it seems. She seems to like us a bit. I think she's OK. I cry.

3

SUMMER
THREE MONTHS OLD
GETTING USED TO IT

Horizontal (Glastonbury Festival
Poetry Diaries)

Cherry Blossom

Rowing Boats and Train Rides

Bashing Breasts

Bite My Thumb

I Lie

3 months old

10 a.m.

It is surreal being back at Glastonbury again, although it is much easier doing poetry gigs with a baby than it was with morning sickness last year.

She is sleeping in a basket by the camper van as me and Dee lie on the grass arguing over whether to take her to Shakira or Snoop Dog. Behind the poets' camping area is Arcadia, a massive sound booth/DJ set where deejays blast out drum'n'bass all night, accompanied by fire rockets every time the bass kicks in. I can't get to sleep because of the noise, and when I finally have it has woken me up the last two nights running. Little One hasn't given a toss and so far has slept through every drum-fire explosion. I think she is so used to Dee's music that to her it's like a lullaby.

Strange how much changes in a year.

Horizontal (Glastonbury Festival Poetry Diaries)

As I lie in the Green Fields with a baby clutched in hands
I tell her tales in softened tones she barely understands
She's three months old and smiling bold
I speak of times twelve months ago

of the same spot
where her mum stopped
and rocked in calmer flows –
In the peaceful palms of Glastonbury
many barely know.

It goes . . .

After King's Cross toilets
after the blue cross
after hands to face
and confused then laughing sobs
I found this spot
In the middle of a field
in the back of a tent
with no one around

After the train journey there
three hours staring at three tests
after the decision face to face was best
and despite itching toes
not to phone him yet
that gave me
three days left.
Alone.
No one knowing but me.
And I found this horizontal haven at Glastonbury

I'd imagined a weekend of no-sleep hopes
Planned for Dizzee, DJ
dancing and dope mornings
Yawning through sunrise

and falling at noon
To new tunes, burnt-out shoes
rave tents and who's who.

I'd planned to be awake at five a.m.
as shakes of drum'n'bass busted up my head
Instead I lay awake at three a.m. repeating in my head the word:
Mum.

Alone, in the tent
I heard the hell-bent screams from Trash City slickers
Drunken footsteps passing me at sunrise
as my heartbeat quickened in
Repetitions:
Mum.

I'd planned to be asleep at ten a.m.
dubstep frets from the night before beating up my head
instead I sat awake at nine a.m.
in morning sickness heat
trod sleepily to the green fields
for caffeine-free teas
collecting white-witch remedies
veggie breakfast melodies
rice and peas and ice-cream.

I'd planned to be on my feet at Glastonbury
dancing drunkenly off-beat at Glastonbury
with eyes closed into the back of me
Instead I lay in chai-tea tents
with food trays resting on my stomach
Staring up at ceilings trying so hard not to vomit

Eating meals on my back
spilling tea sips down my chin
into this horizontal experience of festival living.

That weekend, I saw Glastonbury
lying down
heard the same sounds while
spying sky and clouds
avoiding crowds
instead I lay down peering up above
thinking of the blue line
and trying not to throw up

I saw the real star shows support the stars at night
and the smoke escape paths through stage show lights
I saw three little birds fly over the Black Eyed Peas
and the jazz stage bass shaking the tops of trees
the trapeze artists chatting through the comedian's speech
the gaffer tape repairs and the sound-system leads
I saw the rug-stitched ceilings of the food tent heavens
while I ate my way through to a new world vision
sipping Moroccan mint teas with Thai green noodles
Bean-burger baps and apple strudels.

I was
Confused on the way there
but after three days there
the music that played there
and the flavours they gave there
the colours of ceilings
a focus for breathing
and when the crowds started heaving

the green fields came dreaming
with massage for healing
and herbal brews steaming
with families beaming
and calm babies sleeping
by yoga tent meetings
with mums and dads eating
while children out seeking
and I realised that people are not all the same
and I started feeling OK
Saying 'Mum'.

After King's Cross toilets, after the blues, after hands-to-face
        sobbing and feeling confused, after morning sickness
        tent wakes and star-staring hues, after three days of music
        streaming through tunes
after spices and circus and poetry dos
after getting home and telling my boyfriend the news
after one year on
now I'm vertically tipped

I'm back at the festival
Our first family trip.

What is it about this place? It feels like a magic fairground ride. Last year I was pregnant, this year, I've won tickets to Australia. Two tickets for me and Dee to Australia. The baby's flight is £75. And we're at Glastonbury.

I never thought I would win this: a British Airways competition for people who have been invited to perform or study abroad, to represent their country, but can't afford the flight. It's a good marketing thing for BA, I know that. A way to look 'young' and 'fresh' and get young people sharing the BA name everywhere. You have to get people to vote for you to win. I can handle that. It would still be a dream. Because with a baby, I really can't do a lot of the gigs I'm asked to do. I can't leave her for more than two hours and most event organisers can't pay for me and her and Dee to all go. So someone without a kid will always get the opportunities. So I entered.

Last week, I was seventh in the running out of ten finalists. Then yesterday, on the last day of getting the public to vote, me and Dee looked around. Around a music festival, one of the biggest in the world, with fields and fields of people. Public. And a lot of spare time on our hands.

So yesterday was spent, phone in hand, getting about a thousand people to vote for me online.

'Uh, what? Yeah cool.' [click]

'Do you have a light?' [click]

'Want a spliff?' [click]

'Where am I? Oh, yeah. Sniff.' [click]

'Love you man, sure I can, so much love right now.' [click]

Dee had to have slightly different tactics, to make him 'more approachable' as he puts it. Whether consciously or not, you see people nervous when, as a young black male, he approaches. You see people cross the road, assume he won't have a ticket on a train; he's stopped at customs, checked for drugs, asked for drugs on holidays, stopped by the police more. Anyone who says this structural racist shit is not happening any more just needs just to follow him for a month. It's a really sad way to grow up.

One of the reasons he says he loves having a baby, apart from obviously having the actual baby and being a father, is because for the first time in his life, people in the street smile at him. When he's with her, especially when he has her in a sling, he goes from 'young black male' to 'sling-carrying male' or 'dad'. I think he would like a baby strapped to him for the rest of his life for this reason. It's crap.

So he was only into this if he could carry Little One. So while I walked round approaching strangers sleeping on grassy fields, he walked round getting mobbed by women coo-cooing over our baby (and him) until he butted in and got their votes. And it worked. We got a lot of votes. I went from seventh to first place and we are actually going on a family work trip to gig at the Australian Poetry Slam. We just have to wait for a year so that Little One is a bit older – but not over two years and therefore full price on the flight!

3½ months old

4 p.m.

Bring on the warm days. You are so much more content outside. The cherry tree in the park is like the best baby mobile I've known. A bit of wind and you stare at it for hours. You also sleep better outside, which is slightly annoying but all right now it's warmer.

Really, all the shit that we buy and you are way more contented just lying under a tree watching the branches. Like a gigantic moving mobile. Makes sense really, just wish I'd thought of it before.

Cherry Blossom

The cherry blossom is falling like snow
The swan's nest is guarded, helping them grow
As you lie there, oblivious
Content and eyes closed.

I rock your pram over a stone
Stare at the sparkle on the warm water glow
Brambles and butterflies sway to and fro
As you lie there oblivious
Content and eyes closed.

The sun makes my freckled cheeks show
As you lie there dreaming of daddy's next show
Oblivious, content, peaceful, eyes closed
Unaware of the wonders you'll know.

3¾ months old

I have never been so glad of the World Cup in my life. I mean, I like football, but today I loved football like I've never loved anything.

I've started doing quite a few gigs now and Dee has been driving up and down the country with me so I can feed Little One before going on stage. It is really hard to keep this up, and without him I would have absolutely no chance to be doing it. None. He stands in the corners of poetry venues holding a baby. He has walked her round London streets, held her crying while I finish my set, slept backstage. Mum too. She's been out for dinner at midnight in Chinatown with a three-month-old because, as an under-eighteen, I couldn't bring the baby into Ronnie Scott's Jazz Bar during my gig. A bit annoying that no one told me that until we got to the door that night. So mum and Little One wandered the lights of Chinatown and dozed in the car.

Yesterday I had another gig in London. So we packed up the car and Dee drove.

It was a really shitty journey. Like anything now, the whole day seems to depend on the mood of the small person beside us. This one was terrible. It was hot, the traffic was awful and every time we stopped, Little One screamed her face purple. I sat in the back trying to calm her, wondering why the fuck I was putting everyone through this. I'm sure Dee must've been thinking the same. We couldn't stop anywhere and I ended up feeding her by pulling my seatbelt loose, twisting my body around so I was kneeling on the middle seat with my boob in her mouth, Dee driving seventy miles down the M11. At least she stopped crying. Not sure it's legal to breastfeed like that though.

Eventually, all of us in shitty moods, me feeling like a selfish bitch for wanting to do a badly paid gig in London when we could've stayed home and chilled out, we got to the bar. Parking was tricky. I jumped out to run into the bar. Immediately, I had that feeling, that feeling that something is not right. No chairs were set up, no posters about the gig. The cold blood started pumping through my body with the same sense of panic I had when I was caught stealing sweets from the local village shop or when you try on a dress in a changing room on your own and get stuck in it, head covered, knickers on show. Cold panic. Throat went dry. I walked up to the bar staff and, already knowing the answer, asked if the gig was on.

Tomorrow.

The gig is tomorrow.

The fucking gig is tomorrow.

Why am I doing this? I look out of the bar window. Dee is in the car and Little One is crying. He gives me that 'So what's going on?' look, slightly agitated after the drive. Not only have we wasted the day, but we will have to do this journey again tomorrow. I don't want to tell him this. Not at all. I want to flee. Run. I feel sick.

Dee is getting out of the car with Little One now and I walk up to him.

'It's tomorrow.'

Silence. We stand in the bar.

'Do you want a drink?'

I get him a drink. We're both silent. The football comes on. The World Cup match. Dee sits down.

'If we're here for no sodding reason, I'm watching the match. You're lucky Hollie.' He smiles.

I love football. I fucking love football.

135

4 months old

We went to Wells-next-the-Sea today, played crazy golf with Little One strapped to Dee (he still won) and had fish and chips. Then we went on a rowing boat; a last-minute decision. In the middle of the lake, of course, she started screaming. She wanted fed. I have never been so glad I am able to breastfeed. I feel really lucky today. The sun is shining and so far, I've had no problems with this. My boobs hurt, yes. I feel trapped sometimes, yes. But that's it. It's a blessing, I'm very grateful.

Rowing Boats and Train Rides

In the middle of the night when she wakes up
When we've gone to the park
Or just out for a walk
When I'm round at a friend's
And we want to talk more than I thought we would
When we're stuck on a boat that we can't row so quickly
Or I'm sat on a train and not quite at the city
I don't need to worry about food for her
I don't need firm plans every day that I'm with her
I don't need to go back to the house
To pick up more bottles or another eight ounces

I don't need to sterilise stuff or find somewhere to warm it
I don't have to worry about boiling the water
'Cos I've got everything ready right here in my body
And my boobs are so much easier to carry
Than all that.
I cannot forget them
It's easy to pack them
And if I want to change plans
I don't have to go back for them
I don't need a whole bag for them
I don't need to plan for them
I've got enough to think of already.
Every time I go out there are nappies and bibs
Changes of clothes just in case she is sick
And the idea of having to pack up all this:
bottles, water, formula milk
Worry if it's sterile, find somewhere to heat it
I don't understand why that is more easy
Than boobs.
A bag full of free food prepacked in my body
Nothing to remember, nothing extra to carry
And on top of all that, I do not have the money
To spend on something that's prepared in my body for free.

18 JULY

4 months old

I was reading about the Maldives today, the beautiful island I've only ever seen in postcards. I was Googling 'holidays', daydreaming about having the cash to go there. I found an article about the Maldives. During the elections, it said, breastfeeding mothers who went to vote for the 'wrong' party were targeted by the regime. Their breasts, specifically. Their breastmilk, more specifically. I watched an interview with a woman over there.

Bashing Breasts

We started quite similar
on our way to vote at the polls
ticked our boxes
posted them
went home

but before she could run
he picked up his stick
fingers and fist.
They are trained to hit horizontally.
Push the batons quickly and forcefully.

Under orders, they target mums
striking bruises and scars
to rob them of tongues
and food for their babies
battering breasts
till they are flattened completely.

She sank to the ground
screams stuck in her mouth
and the first time her baby cried out for his feed
his mum dropped to her knees and pleaded

Please—
In my country
breasts are like gold
like votes
like the freedom of speech
washed away by the seas that we see
on postcards of her home

Picture perfect to roam
the Maldives

Where soldiers waited with batons
to bash breasts flat
so babies would starve for
the fact that
their mums voted
Democrat.

4½ months old

She is teething. Sleep has stopped. I'm tired. I have frozen melon skins in the freezer for her to chew on, which seem to help. And I get to eat the melon, so all good. But it must be really shite.

Bite My Thumb

I bite my thumb at your chew toy, mum
Wee on your shite teething ring
As my gums spit broken, swollen skin
Please picture the pain that I'm in

As you lie in your dentist chair, sip antiseptic
A painkiller nation, all I get is to chew
on some plastic
Please!
Are you kidding me?
My thresholds are pushed
Like my skull cap in labour I took all I could
You call me a kid to cover your backs
When your molars come through
– should I give you a chew toy for that?

5 months old

I Lie

My friends don't have kids
and still can't believe I do
'But you,' they say
'Hollie
I can imagine anyone but you.'

So strange to see us with a child
They ask me what it's like
and when I answer them
I lie.
I lie.
I say
'It's fine, hard work but really nice.'
as if those words well describe
I say
'It's tiring but really lovely.
Yeah. Lovely.'

I don't tell them all the times I cry
Tired eyes looking at her, amazed,
to experience every tiny feature of her
fresh canvas face
or that I gaze into daydreams
as she sleeps
because I can't believe it either.
'I'm a mum,' I repeat

I don't tell them that my heart steeps
in heavy breathless attacks
every time I try to leave the room
or that feeding a baby
till they fall asleep on you
is bliss
or that I miss you
as soon as you're asleep

That a warm, tiny palm
pressed against your chest
for security
and a mouth open wide
as the milk stream sends you sleep
is pure beauty

That lips open by a nipple in laughter
and dreaming breaths beside your bedside
and wide eyes waking in the morning
looking round in strange surprise
and smiling when they see your smile
or hear your morning call
is incomparable

That I'd rather die than see her sad
and never had my heartbeats burst before.
that I feel sore when strangers don't smile back at her
and I'd like to hide her in my womb once again
to protect her from the world.

That pride is no description
of watching life before you living
and in the living room
seeing her on him speeding round
and clowning around
and dancing round to reggae beats
and cracking in hysterics
makes me cry again

That it is indescribable
witnessing this small human change.

'What's it like?' they say.
I just smile and say, 'It's strange.
I mean lovely, yeah, but strange.'

4

AUTUMN
SIX MONTHS OLD
SEX AND FEEDING

Embarrassed

Breasts

Breasts – Part Two!

I Would Love To

D.I.L.F

Normal Again

6 months old

I didn't expect to sit on public toilets this much when I had a baby. But I have been. In restaurants, cafés, shopping centres. People go on about the feeding rooms but the one in the local Mothercare is like a stock cupboard that smells of moths. I sit in the dark like a bloody outlaw to feed a baby. The one in John Lewis is better but I'm so tired of running the entire length of town to the top floor, while Little One is crying, just to sit next to babies having their nappies changed. I am tired of the feeding cloths I try to cover her head with. They fall off. Babies move. They kick their legs. I think I have flashed my nipple more times picking up the 'cover cloth' than if I just didn't use it. What a joke.

This is the most tiring thing I have ever done in my life and I live in a country that makes that simple task of feeding your child so they do not die feel bloody criminal. I am tired of this more than anything else that parenthood brings. I have to feed her every few hours so, no, I can't stay at home to do it. Yes, it's awkward when people don't know where to look. *I* don't know where to look sometimes. But I don't know where to look when people snog on the street, or when my friend eats with her mouth open. I feel awkward when I'm asked questions. I feel awkward watching people dance but I don't tell them to stop because it makes me feel awkward. Awkwardness is part of our stupid culture. But feeding a baby? I'M FEEDING A BABY. Why do I feel awkward about it? It is clean, hygienic and it is keeping her alive.

I am so lucky I can do this without mastitis, bleeding, blocks. I can go out without taking bottles or powder, or sterilisers or refills. It is free, that's a big point for me. This is totally free. I have no problems except with our stupid culture. I should think myself bloody lucky. Erica has mastitis. She is a goddamn legend, sitting with cracked nipples trying to get milk out in agony. I don't know if I could cope with that. Thank God we have other options. So I need to woman up about this. It is a blessing, Hollie. You are very lucky. Forget about a few stupid comments.

13 SEPTEMBER

6 months old

2.45 p.m.

I am on a toilet lid. Again. I can smell shit and my baby is asleep. But it's nice to sit down. I feel like a failure. I make excuses that it's good to get space, peace to feed. But truth is, I just feel awkward, when I'm on my own, without Dee, or my mum, or friends. Summertime was bliss. Outdoor feeding. No worry about spills or leaks. I fed at the top of the Wallace Monument for God's sake.

But colder now, so I'm indoors. I have avoided visiting friends with colds, hospitals and any other germ-filled place, in case Little One gets ill. But here I am sitting on the lid of a public toilet feeding a baby in possibly the dirtiest place there is. What the fuck am I doing? But I don't know where else to go. It's raining outside and I'm just shopping, so where do I go?

I should sit on the benches in the shopping centre. I would if Dee was there. Or my mum, or anyone. So why not when I'm on my own? There is a poster on the door, for the Fez Club. A woman dancing in a bikini. And I am on a toilet seat. A woman feeding a baby. I won't do this any more.

I feel terrible – look at you, Little One. You are so bloody beautiful. A tiny human being and I'm giving you your dinner on a toilet seat. Or else with a blanket covering your head so no one can see the fact that you have your lips round my nipple. Welcome to the real world, love;

we find it disgusting to see babies eat here – fancy staying? Want to move somewhere else? Sweden? Me too. What a joke. What a fucking joke. Perhaps you'd prefer it if I let her scream and cry and wail until I get home? I'm hating the world today. I can't believe I'm embarrassed to feed my own baby. What is this shit! My boobs, my baby. People keep telling me to be modest, discreet. *Come on!* I'm not standing on the table swinging my boobs in anyone's face. And anyway, we don't care about boobs. No one told me when I wore low-cut vest tops to be modest. We don't have a problem with boobs at all. We have a problem with babies sucking on nipples, let's be honest here. Who would've known there'd be such a fuss!

Someone asked me why I wanted to feed in cafés last week. I smiled and said, 'I don't. It's just sometimes I want to go to cafés and she may need to be fed there.' For fuck's sake (I didn't say), I don't *want* to feed in a café, I don't leave my flat, take two hours to get the baby ready, pack a baby bag, change her, feed her, step out of the door, she poos, go back inside, change her again, wash poo off her legs, trek into town, just to go to a café to feed her. No, most of the time, I am at home. But sometimes ... just sometimes ... I might want to leave the flat. Is that OK? Sometimes I (and she) want a walk, go to the shops, to work, to the park. Sometimes I have to get a bus or a train. Sometimes I have to take her to work. And yes, I normally feed her first. Who wants to feed their kid on a bus? No one. But babies are not robots, I have not given birth to a robot, last time I checked.

Sometimes she is hungry when I don't expect it. Sometimes I want to leave my house for longer than three hours at a time and now that it is raining more, I will be inside more. Sometimes I don't want to organise my entire life around every feed. I was reading about a mum chucked off a bus. Someone was arguing that it was a natural thing to feed a baby. Someone else said: 'So is poo and wee and sex and we don't do that in public.' People kept comparing it to those things. No one compared it to eating! Or sweating or crying or to other natural functions we *do* do in public. Oh Lord, I'm bored with even thinking about this. I am feeding a child with my own body, everything is going fine and I am saving thousands of pounds doing it. Never in my life did I think that feeding a child would be an issue. Weird, weird place. This is not about boobs. It's about baby nipple-sucking. I wish we could all just admit that.

I will not do this ever again. Not one more dirty-toilet feed. Breathe in. Dee was right:

'Don't worry about it. You're feeding our baby, Hollie, that's all you're doing.'

I'm tired of this. All it boils down to is that people here feel uncomfortable seeing the sucking. Because we have been trained that sucking a nipple is a sexual thing. Which it can be for sure. But our bodies have so many uses. Every inch of our bodies can be sexual. And not. I put a tampon in the same place I have smear tests and sometimes have drawn a hard penis into. I do not confuse the three. They do not feel the same. I do not think I am shagging the tampon or that my boyfriend is doing a swab on me. I use my tongue to kiss and to eat. I don't worry that I am snogging my dinner. I kiss my daughter and my mum and my partner. Those lip to skin touches do not all have the same effect on me. They do not feel the same just because it's the same body part or action. Just as a man flicking his tongue sexily across my nipple and sucking a bit while we both gyrate naked on each other does not have the same effect on me as a baby strapping its lips round my nipple and sucking milk out like its life depends on it (which it does) while I'm sat in my jeans on the couch. Both can feel nice. Both sometimes don't feel nice. But Jesus, if the feel of your baby drinking from your nipple does feel nice – which it bloody well should if you can relax and not feel like a weirdo – it doesn't mean you are turned on by your baby for the same reasons as you would be a lover. Both are intimate. Both are close. But not the same. Argh, fuck this!

I'm sick of pretending I'd rather feed in peace and private just because we are so awkward in this country about bodies and sex and nerves and feelings.

I wish it were summer again. She is so damn lovely. Sorry, kid. I'm an idiot. You don't have to eat on the loo any more. Or in the dark. You can eat where every other human being eats. I'll save the toilets for changing your nappies from now on.

Embarrassed

I thought it was OK
I could understand the reasons
There might be young children, or a nervous man seeing
This small piece of flesh that they weren't quite expecting
So I whispered and tiptoed with nervous discretion
But after six months of her life spent sitting on lids
As she sips on her milk, nostrils sniffing up shit,
Banging her head on toilet-roll dispensers,
I wonder whether these public-loo feeds offend her
'Cos I'm getting tired of discretion and being polite
As my baby's first sips are drowned drenched in shite
I spent the first feeding months of her beautiful life
Feeling nervous and awkward and wanting everything right.
Surrounded by family till I stepped outside the house
It took me eight weeks to get the confidence to go into town
Now the comments around me cut like a knife
as I rush into cubicles feeling nothing like nice
Because I'm giving her milk that's not in a bottle
Wishing the cocaine-generation white powder would topple
I see pyramid-sales pitches across our green globe
and female breasts banned
unless they're out just for show.
And the more I go out, the more I can't stand it
I walk into town, feel surrounded by bandits,
'Cos in this country of billboards covered in tits
And family newsagents' magazines full of it
WHSmith top shelves out for men
– Why then don't you complain about them?
'Cos in this country of billboards covered in tits
And family newsagents' magazines full of it

WHSmith top shelves out for men
I'm getting embarrassed
in case a small flash of flesh might offend

And I don't want to parade this, I'm not trying to make a show
But when I'm told I'd be better just staying at home
And when another mum I know is thrown off a bus
And another one told to get out of the pub
I'm sure the milk-makers love all the fuss
All the cussing and worry and looks of disgust
As another mother turns from nipples to powder
Ashamed or embarrassed by comments around her
As I hold her head up and pull my cardie across
And she sips on the liquor made by everyone's God
I think for God's sake, Jesus drank it
So did Siddhartha
Muhammad
and Moses
and both of their fathers
Ganesh and Shiva and Brighid and Buddha
And I'm sure they weren't doing it sniffing on piss
As their mothers sat embarrassed on cold toilet lids
In a country of billboards covered in tits
In a country of low-cut tops, cleavage and skin
In a country of cloth bags and recycling bins.
And as I desperately try to take all of it in

I hold up her head, I can't get my head round
The anger towards us and not to the sounds
Of lorries off-loading formula milk
Into countries where water runs dripping in filth
In towns where breasts are oases of life

now dried up in two-for-one offers enticed
by labels and logos and gold-standard rights
claiming breastmilk is healthier
powdered and white
packaged and branded and sold at a price
so that nothing is free in this money-fuelled life
which is fine
if you need it or prefer to use bottles
where water is clean and bacteria boiled
but in towns where they drown in pollution and sewage
bottled kids die and they knew that they'd do it.
In towns where pennies are savoured like sweets
We're now paying for one thing that has *always* been free
In towns empty of hospital beds
Babies die, diarrhoea-fuelled – all that, breastmilk would end.
So no more will I sit on these cold toilet lids
No matter how embarrassed I feel as she sips
'Cos in this country of billboards covered in tits
I think
I should try to get used to this.

18 SEPTEMBER

6¼ months old

1 p.m.

Sex

It is now over six months and I'm still not really up for it. I'm starting to feel guilty. I feel like the two top erogenous zones in my body are now no longer erogenous, or at least not nearly as much as they were. Please just touch me somewhere else. Anywhere else. Just, not there. Not my breasts and not my crotch. Neck, back, thighs, arms, shoulders, feet. Any of them. ANYWHERE ELSE.

And it's awkward, I hate telling Dee to get off. To not touch my boobs, but when they're dripping milk and sore and, well – I feel bad now. He's so patient, but I know it must be wearing. Weird for guys. Today you can; not today; today not my boobs; today don't touch anything. It's horrible. Confusing. But I just need my body back and then I'll work it out again. I keep thinking that I don't have time to have sex, but that's not it. We do have time to have sex. I just don't have time to feel sexy. I can't switch on and off like that. My boobs hurt and my mind cannot stop thinking about the fact that at any point Little One may start screaming or crying or just wake up. Sexiness isn't the same as sex. Sex, yeah, you have time to do it. But I don't want to have sex for the sake of it, I want sexy sex. And feeling sexy as a new mum with a new body and a knackered body and mind, and a child in the next room, it's hard.

It's hard, that's all. I'm finding it hard. And a pair of lacy red pants won't solve it. I need a week away, thirty hours' sleep and a full body massage. Neck, back, legs, ankles, feet, shoulders. Anywhere but my boobs.

At the six-week check-up after birth, the nurse looked between my legs and said I'm healing. And then she said, 'You're OK to have sex again.'

'You're OK to have sex again.'

And I thought, 'Fuck you.'

What the nurse *meant* was: 'You can now insert a penis into your vagina without any negative post-birth-related health effects.' That does not mean I'm ready to have sex. That doesn't mean I want to have sex. My vagina is OK, maybe, thanks for that. My head, no. And sex isn't just a penis in a vagina, no matter what Victorian sex education or Hollywood scenes teach us.

And Dee's not a twat and we talk and he jokes all the time, 'Now that the nurse said we can, remember?' And it *is* funny. And I wonder what it's like for women whose partners aren't like him. Abusive partners or partners who feel it's their right to have sex again, despite how the woman feels. I'm annoyed I even feel bad about this, as if at this point I am really meant to be worrying that I'm not being sexual enough when all of this other stuff is going on around me day and night. No wonder people used to commonly separate the partner they had kids with from their lover. Or lovers.

Sometimes I think I'm over-reacting. Then I think it'd be like if a guy had his penis slowly inflated over a period of nine months, then bashed with a hammer for thirty hours till it ripped, then it bled for eight weeks and his nipples swelled, cracked, became baby toys and then on top of the pain and frustration, he felt constantly guilty for not really feeling 'in the mood' while every image from society told him how unsexy his new body and bashed penis was.

But I do feel sorry for him. And I do feel guilty. Because it's been a while now since I knew what the hell was going on. We keep visiting a friend who tells me how horny she was when she was pregnant and how 'she couldn't wait to get back to it' after birth.

'Know what I mean?' she says. I smile and imagine beating her over the head with a wet fish.

My body is not my own any more; it has hands on it all the time and the last thing I want is more hands on me when the baby is resting. But that's shit. I do want his hands on me, I crave them too. But I want to sleep more. A woman told me their relationship became so awkward that she made herself T-shirts so her husband could stop hanging around like a sensual criminal in the bedroom. There were three T-shirts, which said:

'Participatory'
'Non-participatory'
'No'

'Participatory' if she was up for it. 'Non-participatory' if she was up for it but completely exhausted and so sleep-deprived she was unable to move 'so he'd have to do the work on those days'. And then 'No', if she'd had a day of bitten boobs and baby grabs and just a bit too much of her body groped already. Or just didn't want to have sex. She said they both loved it. To be honest, I reckon the T-shirts should be put in the hospital pack rather than the baby lotions and Johnson's offers. And bra vouchers, because mine are all milk-stained. Bras should be on the NHS, with sanitary products and sleep.

Anyway.

Breasts

No one talks about this.
They whisper round it.
With tabooed torchlights
we stumble down it.
I didn't read about it
and I read a lot.
Like writer's block
we stop at breasts.

A naked chest
and my breaths are sickened:
they feed her;
he feels them
and my nerve ends quicken
in panic.
I'm trying to manage the two in one body
I've got two lives each night
and they're both wanting on me.

As we sit down at six, she sips like Siddhartha
My arms heat her belly and her lips sleep in laughter
then after
lights low
I hear Barry White melodies
and step to the next room
where he's waiting so patiently.

From skin to skin baby
to skin to skin man
from staring at innocence
to staring at pants
and it's hard

It's sooooo hard now

to transfer position
from one room to the next in one dim-lit partition.
And I wish I could just split my body in two –
One boob for sex;
the other to feed through.

And they make you feel sick
and they make you feel strange
asking questions like:
'When she's feeding is the sensation the same?'
When her tiny hands tap at the skin on your breast
Of course it's not the same as strokes felt in sex

And we stress that it's strange or it's weird or it's wrong
when from lovely to lover our bodies move on
and my brain took a long time to calm to the notion
that my boyfriend's hands were not planned as imposing

So I lay her to sleep
and wipe off the milk
and step into the next room
for some innocent filth
in the middle of which
her scream jolts me up

And I transform breast once more
between lover
and love.

I don't feel like that poem was totally right. For some days, it is. But actually, for today, I'm not so sure. The ending was sweet. But I think it was sweet because that's how I want to feel. Am I trying to convince myself that I'm happy about these feelings by writing them down like that? I feel a bit of a fraud. Argh. Sometimes it is lovely. Sometimes I don't mind moving constantly between two people who are both equally lovely. But sometimes standing in the hallway between bedrooms unsure which way to move, well . . . sometimes there's a second version of the poem. An extended version. More truthful? I'm not sure.

Breasts – Part Two!

No one talks about this
couples creep around it
lose more sleep
get depressed
or feel distant about it

I didn't read about it
and I read a lot
Like writer's block
We stop at breasts

A naked chest
and my breaths are sickened –
They feed her

He feels them
and my nerve ends quicken
in panic
Trying to manage the two in one body
there are two people each night
and they're both wanting on me

As I sit at six, she sips into calmness
My arms heat her belly
and her lips sleep in laughter
then after, lights low
I hear Barry White melodies
and step to the next room
where he's waiting so patiently

From skin to skin baby straight to
skin to skin man
From staring at innocence
to staring at pants
and it's hard now

It's soooooo hard now

To transfer position
from one room to the next
in one dim-lit partition
and it's been months now
but it's still hard to do
and I wish I could just split this body in two:
One chest for sex
The other to feed through

And they make you feel sick and they make you feel strange
asking stuff like: 'When she's feeding, is the sensation the same?'
When her tiny hands tap at the skin on your breast
of course it's not like stroking in sex
and we stress that it's strange or it's weird or it's wrong
when from lovely to lover our bodies move on
and it's taking me a long time to calm to the notion
that my boyfriend's hands
aren't planned as imposing
and I feel like I'm always repeating this line:
I'm tired, I'm exhausted, I just want some time

and sometimes it seems like my body's not mine
'cos for over a year it's been for someone else
and I don't recognise it
and I don't have the right to it
and she gropes me all day
and as soon as she's sleeping
then he wants to play
and I wonder when I might have some time for myself
'cos I don't have the adult time he has at work
and I don't think he gets that
and he jokes my boobs used to be his
and now they're for her
and I don't think that's fair
because they're mine

THEY ARE ACTUALLY MINE

and they have hands on them all of the time
and sometimes I don't know how much touch I can take
and those are

the reasons I say:
'Don't touch me today
I don't want to be awake.'
'Let me sleep.'
and even speaking that way makes me feel sick with guilt

I know it's hard for you
but this is hard for me too

I love being touched by you
and know that it's just 'cos you care
and you like it when both of our bodies are there
and of course I do too –
Just right now
maybe not quite as much as you do

and it's hard to feel sexy when my top's wet with milk
and it's leaking on you
and I've spent the day being patient
and motherly too
and if we do start to touch
and I love touching you
I know in an hour I'll be in the next room
and if I lay her to sleep and wipe off the milk
and step into our room for some innocent filth
in the middle of it a scream will jolt me up
and I'll transform breast once more between lover and love
from one room to the next all bloody night
when I just want my body back to be mine

I don't want to be touched all the time.

I feel horrible saying it, I know it's all fine
because I love feeding her
and I love feeling you
but right now I think I'll just cry

From one room to the other all bloody night
Back into bed, then into her room,
Sometimes I just stand in the corridor
between the two
watching you
and watching her
and wondering which way to turn
and whether any space will let me sleep

I just wish sometimes no one needed me

and I don't want to feel guilty and tired all the time

I just want a body that's mine.

6½ months old

1 a.m.

I Would Love To

I would love to want to kiss you across your skin each night
I would love to want to talk and eat and drink and laugh and
    dine
I would love to want to share a glass of wine and watch a film
    and lie
entwined till night spins round to sun and watch the reds and
    pinks come up
I would love to want to take you out and spend the night-time
    dancing
And I would love to want to sit and chat and spend the evening
    laughing
And I would love to want to sit with you or lie with you or eat
    with you
and spend the evening time with you, have sex or just relax with
    you
I would love to want to do these things when she's in bed and
    quiet
I would love to want to, but my love,
I'm just too fucking tired.

Nearly 7 months old

Today, I have an epiphany. Watching him. It's the moment I realise I do fancy him a lot, and it's not just because of labour or breastfeeding or the lack of sleep. It's because sexy has changed. That's it. Sexy has changed. I just find different things sexy now. I mean, like, Barry White's music doesn't really do it any more for me now. I hear it and I just think about his nine children and how much work his baby mothers must've put in while he was furthering his own career. Same with Bob Marley: hero, for sure, all good, but who looked after your kids, Bob? Not sexy any more. Not relaxing at the moment.

And nipples, that's a big change.

And when I used to get excited when Dee whispered in my ear, 'Please wait for me, I won't be long, don't go to sleep yet' – now that's just not going to happen. But right now, he is looking so sexy and I find it so sexy when he picks up our baby and gets her dressed and wraps her up in that lovely soft blanket and takes her out of the house. And I can have an hour to myself just to sit and relax. Now *that* is sexy.

And when he says to me: 'No, you sit down, Hollie, you've done enough, I'll make the tea', that is sexy stuff.

And when he comes up to me and whispers in my ear: 'I know I've been to work but just because your work is unpaid and not appreciated by our current government who generally have no idea of childcare in any way whatsoever and therefore ignore it in all policy-making decisions, does not mean that I don't understand that you too have been at work, all day.'

Now that is sexy talk. (He hasn't actually said that last one, but when he does . . . !)

D.I.L.F.

Since I've seen him change a nappy
it seems his penis has grown
Muscles made more pronounced
each time he folds those Babygros
His thighs were pretty buff before
but since he's laid her on the floor
One foot rocking her to sleep
the other touching toes with me
it seems his thighs
Are like three thousand times as juicy now

Since I've seen him push a pram
Cook a meal with kid in hand
Concoct a song to rock-a-byes
Wake to cries with smiling eyes
Pit-stop challenge changing kicks
Cleaning rags of baby sick
Since I've seen him doing this
It seems his bits are twice as big
His neck nape twice as nice to lick
I just have half the time to do it
Since we've had a kid.

10 OCTOBER

Nearly 7 months old

1 p.m.

Dee and Little One are out again. I am on the couch sitting in silence before I try to have a nap

Normal Again

A silent flat
A hot cup of tea
Knowing it's yours for a good fifteen minutes.
Sometimes, that's all I need to feel normal again.

1.10 p.m.

One nice thing about winter coming is that Little One gets to see the stars more. She's still awake when they come out. Well, I don't know if she can actually see them, but we can sit in the evening at the window and watch the stars, it's cosy. And it gets my issues into perspective too. All we need now is a log fire, but I don't think you're allowed them in small flats.

Last night I think I nearly had a whole dream, or at least a dream that wasn't interrupted in the first section, or bit, or whatever dreams are made of. I think she's starting to sleep better now, maybe because it's darker and we're actually inside more in the evenings.

'Don't jinx it, Hollie,' Dee says. 'You know she'll be awake now!' But I can't help getting my hopes up. I cannot remember what it feels like to not be knackered.

5

WINTER
SEVEN MONTHS OLD
BACK TO WORK

Mushy Mummy Baby Brain

First Sips

Don't Touch

Reading to You

Wow!

7½ months old

I started back at work this week. I mean, I've been doing poetry work for a while, but I started back at the office. The day job. Six months' maternity leave added to overtime and holiday leave I'd saved up. All now gone. I'm back. Once again I'll be Education Officer for a small planning charity. Mainly involving sitting at the computer and filling out funding applications.

I have been organising Little One's feeds for the last month and a half so she is eating mashed carrots, banana, whatever, and drinking water while I'm at work. Exciting times. I couldn't pump – I tried but I just couldn't get the knack. I sat for two hours and got one single drop. I don't know what I'm doing wrong. I could've tried again but I honestly can't be arsed. I'd rather just feed. It's so frustrating trying to sit and pump your boob while a baby cries for food next to you. Dee has offered to sit and 'pump me' but that just feels a bit odd. It would be kind of freeing though if I could actually get some milk out. Anyway, she's been loving a bit of mash since she was five months.

I feed her before work and then again straight after I'm home, by which time by boobs are at that swollen, hardened 'touch them anywhere and milk will flood all down my chest like torrents from a broken dam' tension point. I don't have to watch the clock at work, I can work out what time it is from how big my chest is. A bit like those who can navigate their sea voyages with only the stars to light their path, or time their day by the compass of the sun and moon. This is on a similar level to that – by the time I'm nearing Page 3 possibilities, it's likely just an hour till I'm finished. So I've been practising the feeds for the last week and it has worked. I feel chuffed, and slightly annoyed no one has given me a medal for my organisational skills.

The first day back, my boss immediately jokes how 'parched' every-one has been since I haven't been there to make the tea. First thing she says. Funny, hahaha. Less funny because I then go and make the tea for everyone. Still, I laugh a bit. Then Dee calls up at lunchtime because Little One's been screaming at him for two hours and isn't taking any food. He drives over and I feed her. One of my co-workers is a bit unsympathetic with me about it, which annoys me and makes me feel pretty stupid all at once. I feel like I'm doing something wrong again. Like I'm trying to be a pain in the arse here. I'm not trying to be. I'm just trying to work it all out. I'm just trying to work. I realise that legal rights are one thing – actually having the courage to ask for them is another thing altogether. So I feed her as quickly as possible and Dee runs off, apologising. I apologise too, red faced. Then the finance guy we're in the meeting with says, 'My wife's a breastfeeding consultant, it's all good. It's great. This stuff needs to be OK.' Co-worker looks embarrassed. I hug the finance guy tightly in my mind.

That evening Dee apologises again about a hundred times for phon-ing me and bringing Little One to work; says it's so frustrating 'cos there's only so much he can do without boobs. I try to pump again, but I just can't get it to work. Guilt in all directions! I feel terrible as I know other guys are feeding their kids at night. Instead, Dee goes and gets her and puts her on me and she feeds while I sleep. Feeding and sleeping at the same time is a good look!

The next day, it goes fine. She's fine. And work is good. A hot cup of tea (made by someone else today) is good. Working on the computer, doing grown-up things, talking to grown-ups, reading statistics, doing HTML has never felt so great. But I am shattered as well. I would normally be having an afternoon nap now whilst Little One is sleeping, and I realise I can't do that at work. No one told me that when maternity leave is over and you go back to work, your baby doesn't automatically sleep all night now that you can't have a nap. Shit! I joke, but it is really hard to stay awake all night *and* all day.

And last night was bad. Little One was up every hour crying, teething, and the only way to help her fall back to sleep was to read her *The Very Hungry Caterpillar*. The one where a caterpillar hatches, eats some fruit, then some sugary food, swiss cheese, salami, has a belly ache, eats a leaf, cocoons and then turns into a butterfly. And no matter how many times I read it, this part always surprises her. She smiles wide-eyed, then falls asleep.

Not for long though. So I spend the entire night reading the book and watching her fall asleep and then I try to sleep and find myself crying with tiredness and happiness and then being woken up and starting it all again. Eventually I go to bed at seven a.m. and my alarm goes off at eight and I'm at 'work' for nine. Totally knackered, but there. At some point in the morning I can't find my pen. Look around my desk for it. When I ask my colleague if she can see it she laughs knowingly and says I have a 'mushy mummy baby brain' now.

I hear this phrase a lot at baby group. It refers to a non-scientific theory which says that after having a child, a woman's brain turns into mush. Only the women seem to say this. Men at baby group don't say this. I have never heard of 'mushy daddy baby brain'. Men don't say that. Because they don't have it. They call it 'being fucking knackered'. A more accurate description. Well done, dads. For mums, I'd maybe add 'being fucking knackered while dealing with the psychological and physical effects of a complete internal and external body transformation'.

But more often, I hear 'mushy mummy baby brain'. Or just 'forgetful mummy brain' for short.

I find my pen but decide to go on strike for an hour at work and type poems:

Mushy Mummy Baby Brain

I'm a night-time walker, and
a daytime worker now, and
Corridors all smell like beds
Computer screen screensavers flash photos of beaches
As crunching caterpillars munch through the
      desk.

There were ten to begin
One slept
There were nine
Five left, eight fell down
They've cocooned sixty times.

Now beautiful big butterflies emerge from beneath me
As I answer the phone like a drunk on repeat,
'Good afternoon, can I help, who's calling, please?'
They said one went for lunch and then there were three
The meeting's at five, the funders are keen
And the princess is pure 'cos her back felt the pea

On thirty thick mattresses I lie by her bed
My hand on her belly the floor holds my head
My Angel in Cot leaves me tattooed teeth indents
Transforming my skin into tribal-like imprints
I'm in it, *The Jungle Book*, wading through heat
With war-painted patterns two marks on each cheek.

Now my pages are turning
And folder divides
Between nine to five, five to nine, day and night-times

Still the comments come fast, we look older and tired,
That we 'let ourselves go' once we've birthed our first child

We night-time walkers, daytime workers
Smiling in ecstatic pain
And I will beat the next fucker to utter the phrase to me
'Mushy Mummy Brain'.

As history defines us insane and hormonal
Now flittering-minded, unfocused, forgetful
Mental, distracted, absent, hysterical
As if pushing a pushchair now fries intellectual
Strapped in and ready, dummy in lips
Not just the baby, but Mummy and Mrs and Miss
In straitjacket dictionaries these words scratch like lead
Scribbling sexism subjectively fed
As infantile comments sprout from grown men
And I'm told I've lost sense if I lose one placed pen
Put my keys in my pocket and forget that they're there
One missing object held up as female despair

As definitions prepare us for lifelong stupidity
Chronic sleep deprivation labelled mental liquidity
For this unpaid labour they say 'stay-at-home mum'
Painting visions of couches and cookies and school runs
Not called constant carer ready in sleep
Whether you're employed or you're not it's still a full working
        week

And it is bliss and it is heaven and it is amazement defined
And it isn't the start of us losing our minds
And if we seem distracted or preoccupied

It's 'cos our brains never rest and our days stretch to nights
And nights become day as we sit up and read
Hand on her belly as she falls back to sleep
Smiling at her when I just want to weep
And occasional tears do not label me 'weak'

As the last page is turned and I start again one more bedtime
There were ten *very* clever caterpillars,
and now there are nine . . .

8½ months old

Two weeks back at work

I love working. I feel bad saying it, but I do. I don't love my job, but I love working right now. I love coming home to a baby waiting for me and actually excited to see me and me to see her. Really excited because we're not together twenty-four hours any more. I love having something to talk to Dee about other than nappies and how many things I didn't manage to do that I'd planned to do that day. I love hot cups of tea that I can actually drink while they're hot and eating my lunch slower than a bulldozer because I'm not shovelling it in before she cries for me. But most of all, I love that Dee has three days a week with her now and I think we can relate to each other more. And we both agree that work is not *the* work. And 'stay-at-home' parents do not stay at home.

I mean, like, I come home from work and the baby is passed over to me. Because I want to see her and Dee needs a break. I don't. I've been 'at work' all day – drinking hot tea and talking to adults and not having a brain on hyperoverdrive attempting to keep a baby safe and content all day.

He now comes home from 'work' and takes the baby even quicker than he used to because he now knows what it's like – that I might want to wee or sit or remember my own name for a while. Or just not hold my baby for a while, as bad as that might sound. Sometimes, I don't want to hold a baby after a day of holding a baby. Still though, whoever is with the baby still apologises for at least the first ten minutes for all the things they didn't manage to get done.

I start wondering if Swedish couples have better relationships, or at least, resent each other a bit less after having babies. I think I now know who is to blame for post-baby relationship issues too. The government. The UK government, not the Swedish one. The one that gives two weeks' paternity leave so that as soon as you have a baby, the mum and dad are thrown into separate worlds where one thinks the other is getting to stay at home and bond with the baby on a comfy sofa and the other curses the independence and adult life the other still gets. And no one can understand the other's world any more.

And even though relationships between couples are supposed to be a private thing, it's not really a private matter, is it? Two weeks' paternity leave, then he was at work full time again, plus gigging part time, while I was with our baby full time. Full time. More full time I think than any other job in the entire world, bar carers. We were pushed into having two completely different lives, really. I became annoyed he didn't understand exactly how hard this was. He was annoyed he had to go to work at two jobs and not see the baby and still get made to feel bad about it when he was totally exhausted.

When we both started working half and half, I think it eased a bit. I was happier because I was also doing more adult things, talking about subjects other than babies, drinking hot tea. He was happier to be able to help more and not work so much away all the time and see and get to know Little One properly. And have conversations with me about things other than babies. Everything is better for it. Including the orgasms. They are getting increasingly better. It appears that orgasms are stronger and easier to reach when you don't secretly hold a constant undercurrent grudge against your partner. Hard to enjoy touching someone who you secretly think understands bugger all about your life right now.

Well, all I'm saying is I bet Swedish couples get on better after having kids, because the dads pretty much have to take three months' paternity leave, or they lose it. I can't imagine anyone, after six months as a full-time mum, not wanting their partner to know what it's like. I really think it must help relationships. I've got no research to back it up but I think Swedish parents have better orgasms, mainly based on less stifled hate and more shared parental leave. Orgasms; it's all down to politics. Female ones, at least.

8½ months old

Had a meeting with the architects at work today. Lots of talk about their latest projects and their careers. They are all doing really well. One starts on about how he made it as an architect with no help. I wince. Then the younger architect butts in:

'What about your wife? Didn't she raise your four kids so you could have a career, start your practice and become a successful architect? It might have been harder for you to do it from home with all those kids in the way or with childminders' fees.'

I wanted to kiss him. I wanted to snog him right there in the meeting. He stayed in our office afterwards moaning about the architects he deals with. He works part time. His wife works part time. They are both architects. They have three kids. They share the childcare. He has very cool hair too.

9 months old

3.18 a.m.

I can't get over how peaceful babies look after they drink. It washes away all the visions of traumas and tears and screams. So peaceful. Like you would never believe they could be anything but.

First Sips

It's the skin that calmed your first screams
A separation saved in sips
Through frightened lips that slowly calmed
with naked shaking warmed in shaken arms,

As newborn lies in sweated mother's palms
Both scared to death
Together calm

It's a heartbeat synchronised once more
Eyes un-cried in sighs once more
As here becomes a home once more
A haven safe to sleep once more

A bed between the sky and floor
Suspended motion, rocking sores

It's the warmth of chest that shaded eyes
from daylight's break that started cries
It's a shadowed closeness closing nights
As circled arms mimic tight warmth
and the walls of womb and woman

The last attachment baby's given
Sipping nature's methadone
To ease transitions to your own
Your body all alone now
Dragged from inside's peace
to outside's infinity

You feed
as if to merge
with me
once more

11 JANUARY

10 months old

I am in a café. I am not looking after Little One and I am not at the day job (I don't call it work any more because everything is work now). I am just in a café trying to finally organise gigs and update my poetry website. This is the first day I have left her all day with Dee's mum. I am alone with a hot cup of tea. It's frosty outside and I am trying to work but I just keep staring out of the window, watching people walking up and down the street. I haven't done that for a long time. I feel free. No one here knows I have a baby. No one knows I'm a mum, it's weird. I feel like I should tell them. I feel good, though (after crying in the car all the way here). But really, for nearly a year I have been mum or at work, day job or freelance job. Mum or at work. Girlfriend, mum, at work. Not *me*. To remember what things I think about when I'm in a café with a hot cup of tea. Out of the flat. On my own. All the things I used to take for granted. Now they are like magic moments in a new, old world I can almost remember.

Little One is grabbing everything at the moment. It is really peaceful sitting down somewhere and not worrying about people getting annoyed by crying or screaming or grabbing. I look at the table – sharp corners, a boiling-hot drink, stairs close by. But she's not here, I don't have to eye out all the hazards today. She is an explorer now and I love watching her, but the more I see her try to feel for things, the more I notice how much kids constantly get told to stop touching stuff, I

imagine if it was our sight that got picked on instead – parents shouting
'Stop looking at that!' Wanting to touch things is as normal as wanting
to see and hear things – it's amazing how much we stop kids doing it.
Unfairly so, unless they're about to hurt themselves or break some-
thing, of course. I remember when I worked in a clothes shop while
I was studying. Kids dragged along on Saturdays, desperate to play
in the jeans rack. We didn't mind at all, but every time they touched
something they were scolded.

I remember as a kid playing in the massive roll-up tubes in the carpet
shop. It was the best playground I've ever been to. And now, on my
own, hands around a warm mug of tea, just looking out of the window,
remembering what peace and quiet and independent thought feels like.

Don't Touch

Now our fingertips sit frigid
Craving to stretch out
Nerve endings palpitate
Longing to let out

Stimulation teases us
As parents shout
'Don't touch!'
And babies' ready fingertips
Swing below in huff

Toddlers thrilled by shelves and hangers
In shops full of shapes and games
Stretch arm to hand, then sudden bangs –
'Don't touch!'
Comes screamed again

Their fingers cry, though eyes stay dry
Fingertips stick cheeks and sigh
Place palm to face in aching 'Whys?'
As evolution lies denied

Then five years old, fingers crave
To dig, to burrow soily graves
To feel the earth and dampened grass
From tip to lip, a certain path!
And just as skin tips touch the dirt
Oh, joy of joys, to feel the world
A tight-grip fist pulls back the arm
As fingers cry in false alarm
Thrust back to gloves, oh boring warmth!
Frustrated fists prepare for war!
Let earth be quaked by stamping feet
The only link to what's beneath

Now thirteen years old, it's even meaner
As fingers frump in disbelief
Tongue can taste and eyes can see
But fingertips lie lost in dreams
Of cotton buds or pots of honey
Through hairs or grass or cold-coin monies
To drag like nails on blackboard skin
To tickle soles or rough-ride shins
As showers rain like morphine drops
And fingertips rub hair in sobs
For more and longer rubbing times
Like crack cocaine in shampoo lines.

By twenty-nine the twitch begins
Nerves sit back in stifled slings
As fingers tap on plastic keys
For jobs that offer no relief
These deadened tips on deader surface
Tap away with no set purpose
Waves of nauseated nothing
We tip-tap on through plastic touching

And now
So little is felt
not food nor fabrics
Internet shops killed that practice.
Now arms to sides by fifty-five.
As sixty-nine is skipped and dry
Inside a TV lies ahead
and fingertips sit starved, unfed
A kitten's fur the only life
As strokes regain the fingers' rights
Apart from those it's keys and buttons
Remote controls and TV stations
Telephones and keyboard taps
China cups and paper bags

Then once a month the visit comes
Grandma waits with bated lungs
A hug so hard it peels my skin
As fingertips dig out my ribs
Five minutes in, my chest to hers
I hear her finger kittens purr
She hasn't had a hug for weeks
'Since Granddad died,' she says to me

So fingers now are feeling starved
We sink our sorrow in warm-filled baths
Massage culture – not here thanks
From baby age we train our hands

Now my ten-month-old looks up and stands
Palms pressed onto my legs like clamps
Staggering in practised grabs
Around my Grandma's shoes and bags
My kid's hands grope like opened dreams
She wants to feel as much as see

Until:
'Don't touch!'

My Grandma screams.

10½ months old

7.40 p.m.

New bedtime routine: I read to her. I put her to sleep. I sit by her bed and read my own book for half an hour while she drifts off. Sometimes I read it out loud. Bliss. Half an hour to sit by myself and read. If I had to do bedtime every night I'm not sure it'd be as amazing. I think I'd resent it a bit, to miss out on evening time every night. It's such a brilliant time of day, as the sun sets and the lounge lights up with gloaming glows. I don't want to miss that time of day. It also makes me sleepy doing bedtime and I don't want to be sleepy every night at seven. But every other night is bliss. Dee does the same. except on his nights he shuts himself in her room and watches football as she dozes off.

This week I've been reading *Lady Chatterley's Lover* out loud to her. Dee walks in just as I am describing the soft brown blanket that the gardener lays the lady down on in the hut by the chickens. 'What the fuck are you reading to my child?!' I laugh. She looks pretty content with it though. Me too.

Reading to You

I've had some beautiful nights in my life –
sleepovers sneaking downstairs to the fridge

tiptoes with stomachs of bubbling giggles
and wrappers of Snickers and Magnums and dribbles

Some beautiful nights in my life –
on clifftops in sand dunes
on beaches with rave tunes and full moons and new friends
and neon and old scents and crap tents and butt ends
from haze-making grasses and pipes

I've had some beautiful nights in my life –
in beds and on couches
on Sundays just lounging
with comfort and calmness
and arms wrapped around me
and popcorn sounds drowning out
crunching through films
that flash me ideas
till my brain bursts
excitedly hatching up plans

I've had some beautiful nights
in my life

but sitting here
as the night falls
reading to you
as you point to the cow
and I attempt at a moo
and you laugh
and I do it again just for you
and the rain's pouring down
and the sound makes you calm

and your eyelids start sinking
and you battle them not to –
moulded into my arms
and that warm patch of skin
that spreads from your cheek
through your baby-wise grin
and I read to you softly
as your adrenalin gives
and I watch as you sink past that magical gate
turn-point between falling asleep from awake

Of all my nights and the stars I've walked through
Of all of the nights and the parties I've been to
I've had no greater night-times than reading to you
till you sleep
open-mouthed
ear on my arm
heart to my heart
with a laugh
as you drift into dreams
and I finish the book
though I know
you're already asleep

I stare at your face
in the still, silent room

The best nights of my life
have been reading to you.

9 p.m.

I took down the full-length mirror in our flat the week Little One was born. I didn't want to see my body. I was totally freaked out by the feel of it, by what it was doing, and I didn't want to see it. It's an awful thing not to want to see your own body. It's the single thing you own in this world. The only possession you really have in any way. And mine works really well. It's a good, brilliant body. I felt awful to shun it, especially after it had just given birth to a magnificent new human being. But I guess that's how we're made to feel. All the get-back-into-shape pictures. The *Daily Mail* ran an article the other week about 'Yummy Mummies with No Tummy'. New mums that are still 'fit' – as in hot-fit. I know it is absolute bullshit, this stuff, but it is really, really hard to get it out of your brain. Really hard. It helps sales of skin cream too much, perhaps. Or would make women feel too brilliant, maybe, if we actually said, 'Fuck me, body, well fucking done, that was hard. Check out your battle wounds. Here's your medal from the Queen. She gets one and all.'

So I took the mirror down. Crying as I did so. Cut in two between my head and my skin, the one apologising to the other. Ten months later, it's up again. Solely because I got sick of not being able to see outfits in full length when I was going out somewhere. Also, I guess, I'm slowly starting to get used to the new look. Slowly.

So I put up the mirror.

As soon as I'd put it up, Little One crawled up to it, then hauled herself up and stood in front of it. She doesn't like clothes at the minute. She prefers to be naked at all times, so she was naked. She looked at herself. I realised she hadn't seen her own body since she was born. Ever, I mean. My fault. She looked at her belly, her bum, her legs and giggled. She touched her belly. Then she started to bounce on her knees and began applauding herself, smiling. Applauded her brilliant naked flesh. Maybe I should try to do the same. I will. Not right now though.

Wow!

My body is amazing

I can almost hear her saying it
as she stands naked at the mirror
hands clapping in applause to it

She's naked, bold and proud
her mouth open wide and round, like

Wow!
My body is amazing

Near one year old and loving it
full belly sticking out
thighs like mini tyre towers
and when she looks at her reflection
she always shouts out loud like

Wow!
This body is soooooo great

Gazing down now
I try to do the same –
ignore the plastic advert spreads
that pass me on the way
I say 'My body is amazing'
despite what some might say
I say 'My body is amazing'
despite the claims you make

The nip-and-tuck and cuts and sucks that fill my walk to work
     each day
Enhancement ads and happiness will only come with curves *this*
     way

and if I lay in front of you today
clothes dropped to the floor
you'd prescribe me what I could have less of
and what I should want more of

A tick box of what could be chopped off
with red pen ready hand aside
your eyes deciding what to slice
from lips to cheeks to bum to thighs

The lines below my eyes, you say
I ought to peel or pull away
my breasts will start to sag one day
that breastfed baby there to blame
She came into the world you say
that's great
but now behold your face
your saggy stomach, baggy eyes
stretch-mark stripes
You look and sigh:

My eyes, tighten
My legs, inject
My thighs, cut back
My head, perfect
My stomach, flatten
My breasts, enhance

Don't smile too much
Oh God, don't laugh

As you mark me like a canvas page in circled bouts of red
I feel the need to tell you, you might praise this skin instead

'Cos as you chat about correction
your plucking, cuts and lasers
briefcase stuffed with time relapses
scalpel-led erasers
I take up your red pen to my cheeks
and mark two stripes on either side
a naked painted warrior
could be a sorer sight for eyes 'cos
I am ready for your battles now
my body's felt the worst
No scalpel-cut intense
as that last damn push of
         birth
and I have learnt with awed amazement
what my body brave can do
and now I'm marked like tribal tattoos
with the tales my flesh went through

But those stripes that line my 'saggy' stomach
mark me
like gold
and the folds by my eyes tell a tale just as bold
My laughter lines are getting deeper now
because I smile twice as much
so if you palm-read these first 'wrinkles'
my life would light *up*

The official position is that smoothness is queen
but without any lines there's no reading between them

A storybook is opening
my life has just begun
and once upon never plays
if I cling to line one
as you try to cover the living I've done
as a human, a woman, and now
as a mum

But your red pen can't rub out the nights I've not slept
the parts that I've bled
or the laughter I've wept
the baby I held in a stomach that stretched
the breasts that got heavy so baby was fed
the parties I've had out
the sleep I've missed out on
the dinners I've stuffed down my throat like a python
as you pile on the pressure to cover my life
I wonder what the hell is so wrong with your sight

If my mind and my memory can tell you my tales
then why can my body not tell them as well?

as our babies stand naked
applauding their skin
I can't wait for their lives
and their lines
to begin.

11 months old

I have a hangover. My first official hangover in nearly two years. I now realise that having a hangover and a small child are not compatible. Next time, I will only go out for a birthday drink if I can find someone who will babysit while we are out, and the next morning when I need to catch up on the sleep and lie in bed eating potato waffles and cheese. Otherwise, this is just not worth it. She's so cute. I'm so hungover and tired. Get up. Six a.m. Be sick. Play.

Lesson learnt.

6

SPRING
ONE YEAR OLD
A TODDLER

Nearly 1 year old

I am having quite a lot of fun saying 'She's OK at it' when asked questions by other parents. Or even 'No, she's not very good at that.' My entire belly swells up with silent laughter. The email update sent me a chart today about the stages babies will be at if they are 'behind', 'average', 'advanced'. And that was that. I finally decided to unsubscribe. We're obsessed. I don't want to focus on these things. I want to play with my kid. But I love giving negative answers. People are pretty competitive about this stuff.

'Is yours talking yet? What was her first word?'

'No,' I say, 'she's not really saying much.'

'Has she taken any steps?'

'Yeah, but a bit wobbly, not on her own,' I say.

And I don't mean it; obviously I feel a bit mean but I cannot handle the boasting. Baby boasting, it's crazy. I don't want to do it, though I'm sure I've fallen into it. But I am trying hard not to.

'I think she's pretty average at that' is my most common response. And the awkwardness it produces is jokes.

They are babies. But they are all different human beings.

Mine's pretty good at crying at three a.m., though. Better than yours is, I reckon.

The League-table Toddlers

It's the fiftieth time that I've read you this book
and you still get excited with each turn of the page
as if you never remember that those ten crunching caterpillars
will turn into nine if one of them stays

You just gape at my words, completely amazed
your mouth making wow shapes 'cos now there are eight
and as I turn the last page, your breath is taken away
at the miracle finish of butterfly states

In their cushioned cocoons our babies all wait
dreaming of milk streams and breathing and space
Now proud parents gaze at their new babies' faces
and miracle nipples are hunted and grazed

But barely weeks on and we're upping the pace
as play-group parade already takes place
Us parents lined up for the league-table races
the starting fire sounds and the boasts are away

'Mine's very well advanced for her months
She's already crawling and knows the word "Mum"'
'Baby food, nah, she's on burgers and buns
before she could crawl, she started to run
Doesn't yours?' we say
'Doesn't your baby sleep through the night now?
String consonant sounds in sentence-like lines now?'
Now sleep deprivation is nothing compared to this
emails of milestones and marker-point tick lists

But in ignorant bliss you lie naked in bed
and I whisper to you that I couldn't care less
I just stare at your body in still disbelief
thankful for those things you are not going to be

Like standing in school with blue stockings high
ruptured by canes and angry slapped sighs
as into your face signs push words you can't read
that this is no place for girls
so go home, clean and breed

In streets you won't march, past parliament laughs
as you fight just to vote, suffragettes and burnt bras
Your arms won't be tied up in straitjacket claims
your defiance defined as newly insane
hysteria cut out by Freudian claims
as white-coated men come to take you away

You won't pay for your mind by callings to drown you
as crowds surround you calling they found you
third-nipple claims made as the public ungown you
councillors hunting for witch women round you

As you lie I think back to those babies who once lay
fat cheeks pressed to pillows, snoring away
all those chubby-thighed babies and softening curls
who learnt to stand up and then never stood still
who threw off the Babygros and marched into towns
so that one day you'll march into school and sit down
who learnt to walk forward and never turned round
who learnt to speak up and then never looked down

As we pressure ourselves in league-table fights
I wonder if Mother Teresa slept through the night
whether Gandhi crawled first or went straight into walking
whether Rosa Parks spoke before others were talking
whether Emmeline Pankhurst used a bottle to sleep
if Nelson Mandela sucked a dummy for peace

and I smile like I care as I listen to those
desperate for babies to get up and grow

then I stare at your eyelids, sheltering dreams
and smile for those things you are not going to be.

So please remember my dumpling I could not care less
whether your stage is an average, an advanced or a best

Let your legs rest a little
roll around a while more
save your words for a rainy day
and chill on the floor

So when you finally stand up
you won't be pushed down
and when you take your first steps
you'll step well and walk proud
stick that fat belly out
scream out and yelp
'cos there is a world full of babies
that still need your help.

Very nearly 1 year old

She walked. That's it. She walked. First steps on her own. I am more chuffed than when I got picked as rounders captain at school, and I was really bloody excited then. We won the county championship. I was backstop. It was really, really good. I really miss playing rounders. It's far too underrated as a sport. It's like cricket, but actually fun, with fewer people in straw hats saying 'spiffing'. Right now though, I'm more chuffed than all of that.

This week has been great. I'm in Mons, Belgium, on a poetry residency, working with other poets from the UK, Portugal, France and Belgium to write a show. It lasts two weeks. The only reason I could do it is because not only Dee but my mum as well came over for different amounts of time to help. Without them, I couldn't do any of this. Nothing. It has been bloody tiring but so damn exciting. The only gripe of the week has been when other poets have complained about being tired. Now, don't get me wrong, of course you can be tired. But that doesn't stop me wanting to scream pretty loudly into my open palms and blurt out 'FUCK RIGHT OFF, YOU'RE NOT FUCKING TIRED, YOU HAVE NO SODDING IDEA WHAT THE CONCEPT OF TIREDNESS EVEN MEANS!'

I don't normally feel this way. I remember before I was pregnant, a work colleague who had a baby used to shoosh me every time I mentioned I was sleepy. She used to fume with anger at the mention of anyone without children being tired in any way whatsoever. I used to forget this office rule and roll in moaning about getting no sleep and watch her face morph from a very funny and brilliant friend into that of a potential killer in two seconds flat. Although I do get it now, I swore I wouldn't do that to other people 'cos it used to piss me off a treat. People without kids can have insomnia, sleep problems, stress, whatever. Or just be tired. And some people with kids get plenty of sleep. But when it's a group of poets who have been sitting on their arses all day poncing about (I don't want to be insulting, but it feels a little like this at times) with poetry and words on a residency in Belgium. Nah mate, sorry. Shut the fuck up. Even with a child to feed every five hours, even with about four hours of interrupted sleep a night and five a.m. wake-ups, I'm still finding this residency an easy job. Talking, writing poems and reading them to others. Please. It's bliss. It's like a holiday writing retreat.

Maybe I just don't take this art form seriously enough. I know that words are not a passion to me as much as to the others. I mean they *are* a passion, but I don't hunt for the right phrase or sound or metaphor so much. I just take a piece of paper and lash out my thoughts onto it. For some people, the skill of forming and crafting poetry is essential. For me, less so. I would like to care more. But when I have a baby with me, a new life that I have to sustain, that came from my body into the world and relies on me to keep it alive, it's hard to take words on a page more seriously than that.

On the morning of the first day, we were all asked to write one poem based on the theme of supermarket products. We were given ten hours. Ten hours for one poem! Told to come back after five hours just to get a sense of whether ten hours would be long enough for the task. Ten hours! For a practice poem! I realise I've been rushing my work to shit!

When we met back up after five of those hours, one of the poets said they had thought of the first sentence, but wanted to get it perfect. Everyone nodded, like that was normal. Sometimes I can't believe these things. My jaw almost dropped to the floor. I think I'm too practical. Or maybe it's an English thing. Michelle Madsen, the other poet there from England, had a similar open-mouthed reaction. If I'm told to do something, I do it. Quickly. Rushed, probably. But five hours on one bloody sentence? How perfect can it get? As I said, this job is easy. Maybe not easy. Just not tenuous. That was a good word. Tenuous. It's an exciting job too. A bloody pleasure and privilege to do. I am really, really privileged to be here. What it is not is tiring. I will pass my screaming baby to the next person who says that and see how much writing they manage to do. Don't be bitter, Hollie. It's not their fault they didn't have a baby. And their poems will be much better.

Back to the miracle steps.

Dee and Mum and me are in a café eating *frites* – which in Belgium taste like a cross between the best Scottish chip supper and posh French skinny fries merged together in a vat of crispy duck fat and gold fairy dust. We are in the café because I took an hour to write the supermarket poem and then went for lunch, not sure what else to do. As we are talking, Little One suddenly toddles away from us down a cobbled backstreet pavement – on her own. I have no words for my excitement at this. Firstly, because for the last few months I have almost permanently fucked up my back by walking behind her holding her hands, my own body hunched over hers. Dee too. Hunchbacks together. Secondly, well, because I really love her and she just took her first steps in front of me, Dee and my mum. And that's brilliant. And I'm gushy.

The funny thing is, I think she had to wait till it was just our family there to do it. I've always had a bit of a weakness for French, especially when spoken by a deep-voiced human with a penis. It's a genetic weakness inherited from Gaga, my mum's mum. There are two deep-voiced Belgian men on the residency and every time I am walking round the square with Little One and they come over and speak to her – in French, they can't speak English, so I don't know what the effect of just the accent would be – her knees buckle almost immediately and she tumbles to the ground. Every single time. Genetic, that's all I'm saying. Dee doesn't quite believe the science, but . . .

Now, with only our dull English and Scottish accents around her, she is walking. She is walking and smiling and totally in awe of her own greatness as she steps. And steps again. And I melt. My heart has turned to jelly. Not even wobbly set jelly, no – the stage before: before it goes in the fridge, when it is boiling hot and sweet and stolen in dipped spoonfuls and quick sips before Mum catches you and says 'if you drink it all, there'll be nothing left to make the jelly with' and you don't really care because that hot liquid jelly tastes so bloody good anyway. That is my heart.

Watching that first toddle has made me think about life a lot. There's a poem by an Irish-based American poet called Erin Fornoff, with the line 'Think about the last time you did something for the very first time.' I love that. It is perfect for those first steps. Every time I re-picture the utter passion and thrill and belief in herself that shone through her face with those first lone paces, or her first words, or the first taste of a new flavour, I think of that poem.

Watching her eat her first bites of watermelon and pear was similar. Watching her eyes beam and the juice run down her chin as she guzzled through the flesh of those fruits was probably as close to some sort of God as I've ever felt in my life. Realising this stuff is here – grown by magic, full of sunshine and rain and juice and loved with every first bite by this small human seedling. And now her legs are doing their thing. And the ecstasy is there in her face again, pear juice dripping down my mind as I watch.

We always equate that sense of thrill, of novelty, to children, because they learn so many new things all the time and very quickly, at once. But we could too, we just stop bothering. Why do we stop bothering to learn new things? Why do we start to become embarrassed to do new things? I'm only approaching thirty and already I hear people my age saying they're too old to start something or learn or take up a new hobby. What are we doing to ourselves? What are we so scared of? Why are we so embarrassed to scoot or skip down streets or dance in the rain or . . . anything that's fun and free.

I think about the first time I read a poem out loud in the Poetry Café in London. For a whole year before that I would walk past that place each week and never go in. Look through the window, hand almost to the door handle, then buckle and walk away, because I was scared I wouldn't fit in or that people would laugh at me or I would go to the wrong place or say or do the wrong thing.

Then another year of watching other people read in the café before I stood up and read my own poem. What was I so scared of?

I think of all the new things I've done in my twenties; the first time I had sober sex, fell in love; the first time I read out a poem; spoke to someone in a bit of badly learnt Spanish and realised they understood; the first time I stood on a surf board and caught a wave (then fell off and cut my knees open); the first time I gave birth or held a baby and realised 'Fucking hell, I can do this, I can actually do it.' Even watching a new film, or discovering a new band. It is so fucking exciting. I wonder what other things I can do.

Watching her face light up as she wobbled across the cobbled street was magic. But it is a magic that doesn't have to be reserved for children. I think I've experienced a lot. But given all the things I can do and have done, there will always be much more that I cannot do and have not done. If I live till I'm a hundred and do something new every week, the world will still outdo me a million times over. I find it amazing that some people seem to stop at my age – like they've learnt what they wanna know, done what they wanna do and that's it. Settled. Watch TV. Eat. Sleep. Repeat.

The world is so big and I am so stupid and unknowledgeable and unable to do most things it has on offer. I make a pact. Don't be embarrassed to try things, Hollie. Take a few lone steps away from your comfort zones down cobbled back alleys, even if they seem filled with shadows and people who speak a different language that makes your knees topple at the deep-voiced sound of it. In fact, *especially* if they seem filled with shadows and deep-voiced foreign sounds. Don't ever stop doing that. Don't ever stop learning to walk for the first time. Don't ever stop believing you can.

I'm learning a lot from this small child. I hope I can teach her as much as she's taught me already.

30 MARCH

Mother's Day – 1 year old

We took our mums out for dinner today to say thank you.

Thank you, for allowing us to work.

Thank you, for letting us have a night to have a date with each other sometimes.

Thank you, for coming up every Sunday just so we can have a few hours' sleep.

Thank you for looking after Little One every Tuesday despite her screams and tears and yells.

Thank you, thank you, thank you, thank you.

I cannot describe what a lot of thanks they deserve. I keep thinking of my mum these days. She raised two kids. Her entire family still in Scotland and so had no regular help around like I have. No Sunday visits like I get. No break. Ever. My dad leaving early and working late most nights to set up a business; playing golf or hockey at the week-ends because he needed some 'me time' after a hard week at work. If Dee came back and said he was going to go out Saturday and Sunday because he needed some 'me time', I swear to God I'd sob, then cut off his feet. I'm not saying it's not hard. My dad worked hard. Really hard, to earn for his family. I get that. I know my life is easier and better because of it. He had stress and travel and motorway queues and bleak office space on a Slough trading estate. He missed out on seeing a lot of the great stuff my mum saw.

But 'me time' at the weekends for the parent out at work and not the parent looking after the kids – no fucking way. My mum had no days away from us. Not one day to be herself. I can't imagine how hard that was. I bet she never asked for one, either. That's a guilt thing, for sure. I get that. If I ask for someone to watch Little One so I can work, I feel fine. But even the *idea* of asking for help so I can just relax – I find that really hard. I don't know how anyone can ask for it every weekend. Or just assume they have a right to it. I couldn't. I should, but I'd feel terrible. Dee doesn't, either. We both feel guilty about asking for some free time. But at least we both do, I guess!

I don't think anyone can understand the psychological effects of that sense of loss and gain all at once. Gain of a beautiful human, of love and indescribable heart-wrenching joy. Loss of yourself. Of the hobbies and passions and ambitions and outings that just belonged to you. 'Me time' is like gold dust to me. Like oxygen. Like, I-am-not-losing-my-own-personality-or-my-mind-and-feel-like-a-normal-person-again potion. And both parents deserve it. I get it at work now. But that's not proper space away. I also have Dee and our mums to thank for getting some more of it. And I am still knackered. I still sometimes feel like punching a wall or locking myself in the bathroom just to scream or cry from frustration, tiredness, the fact that I have been so patient all day to the ends of my human patience limitations. 'Me time'. It is invaluable to the mental state of parents worldwide. Not one day away from us in five years, Mum. Damn. And now you are looking after my child once a week too on top of a sixty-hour working week. But you say that's because you want to. I hope so.

Thank you. Especially thank you for forcing it on me. Not waiting till I asked. Just saying, I'm coming to babysit. Go out. Go to sleep. Take time off. I need that to be forced on me or the guilt is too much. Thank you. I need people to say 'no, we don't want you to come to the park with us, stay at home'. If you don't say that, I will guiltily stick on my coat and wellies every time.

Oh, and Mum, sorry for waking you up after you'd worked nights at the hospital. Really sorry about that. I didn't really get how tired you were. I just wanted to chat and show you my new cartwheels. I didn't even know what 'night shift' meant.

I realise there are granddads out there who help with their grand-kids too and I love seeing that. But at the moment, with us, it's the grandmas that take their own time to help us out. Maybe one day the granddads will too. I hope so. I think they will. I think my dad would be excellent. He's so good with kids. He's so funny. I can't wait till he realises that. I think both our dads would enjoy being a granddad more if they did more. Maybe. For now they seem to be happy taking the credit for the work and time the grandmas are putting in. Which is a fucking lot.

Grandmas and Bees

Is it 'cos they don't wear suits and shirts
Is it 'cos they don't get paid for their work
That we don't give a shit about bees?

Is it 'cos they don't wear suits and shirts
Is it 'cos they don't get paid for their work
That we don't give a shit about grannies?

Is it 'cos they both like lavender smells?
Is it 'cos their trade isn't named that well?
Is it 'cos neither rides on the rush-hour swell
That we don't give a shit about them?

We look at them both like cute little pets
Grannies and bees, ladies and insects

Knitting and fussing and buzzing around
Making cakes, making honey, no money, no sound.

They say 'Old nagging grandmas and plump bumble bees'
– propping up the foundation of worldwide economies
Amongst flowers and pollen and babies they lurk
So our seeds turn to food and our parents can work.

Is it 'cos they do it without any fuss
Is it 'cos they don't travel rush hour with us
Is it 'cos they do it no money, more love
That we sweep their economies under the rug?

Grandmas and bees, our dear unpaid labourers,
Agricultural keystones and job-market saviours,
If we worked out the money they make for this land
We might start to give them a hand.

10 APRIL

1 year 1 month

I'm finally making a few local 'parent friends'. It feels really good. It's really nice going to other people's houses and hanging out with other parents. It can be pretty lonely otherwise. Really lonely sometimes being with a baby all day. Although the first time at a new friend's house makes me feel like I'm five again, nervously sipping tea and hoping we get on all right.

When I moved into our flat I remember being so worried that I had no friends around. Dee is surrounded by people he knows since school. Everyone I went to uni with here has moved away and my friends are scattered all over the country now. When I told friends I was pregnant one of the main things they said was how I'd probably make loads of great friends now – my mum has three really close mates she met when she was pregnant or through baby groups. Their kids – Jodie and Caroline – are still two of my closest friends. So I had this really strong idea that when I had Little One, when I was pregnant even, I'd go to these classes and hit it off with other mums, then to baby groups and form a group of really close local friends. But that hasn't really happened. No one's fault. Just hasn't happened.

Sometimes in my head I assume that everyone is doing better than I am: that they are all totally cool and together and never ever want to scream at their kids or lock themselves in the bathroom and cry for the night. I worry about inviting people to the flat in case it's not as big or good or neat or tidy as theirs. I think it's that same bullshit attitude I got from the beach-walking pregnancy magazines and the pregnancy-announcement catalogue couple: the idea that everyone but me lives in immaculate white-linen-draped houses with a white sofa from Habitat, a husband and two Golden Retrievers. And a beach house. And a kitchen shining like the smug-lined white hell-hole of Annabel Karmel books.

But that's rubbish and I'm glad that I've now broken that feeling by just inviting people over. Seeing other people's houses has been really good too. Not in a nosy way, just to realise that everyone's stressing about the mess, the toys, the piles of clothes to wash and whether everyone else is more together than they are. I should've done this a lot sooner. There are some really great people round here.

Stuff

We started quite similar
Three parents in awe
watching with pride as they crawl on the floor
as they learn how to walk
and they learn how to fall
and we realise the reason this isn't quite so hard
any more

Now we're going out more and visiting friends
and watching our kids as they begin to pretend
making make-believe men out of teddies
and tents out of sheets
and ships out of mugs

jumping in puddles of mud
passing us teacups of air
pulling our hair
and playing with sticks

and sometimes I wish that reality just stayed like this
and sometimes I think if we all played like kids
I don't think we would be so depressed.

'Cos we started quite similar
all playing and stares
only difference
their front room is still almost bare
and mine's in between
and his is fuller than I've ever seen
toys line each side like a fairground machine
the cot has five speeds
and the pram's a Mercedes
and I worried too much about
our different status
but the babies they all sit
ignoring the grading
ignoring the toys
and biting their toes
and I realise the shopping lists we're handed are gross
that we don't need the stuff that they tell us to buy

and now it seems no great surprise
after almost one year on
that our babies couldn't give a toss
what shop we buy their clothes from
or whose house has more brands

or the design of their prams
as long as they can trust the hands that push them

and as I watch them I wonder why these scams are allowed
why we should feel any more proud if our highchair's the best
    one
and our nursery borders look prettier than the next one
and sometimes I wonder what the point of the fuss is
and sometimes I wonder what all of the stuff is
and right now I think we can learn more from them
than they do from us

as we all sit on cushions
and pretend to drive buses all day

'Cos we all play the same
and we all smile the same
at the end of each day
and we all cry the same
when it's not going OK.

We all start so similar
playing like this
and it isn't a myth that the box
is often more fun than the gift
and right now I can't imagine life
getting much better than this
so good to know other parents and kids
and that all the distraction ignores the fact that

after sleep and food, safety, protection
exploring the world and avoiding rejection

that it really doesn't get much more fun
than bubbles and slides
walking in parks and riding a bike
kicking leaf piles in Autumn
watching blossom in Spring
banging a spoon as hard as you can
stealing a kiss
or getting a hug

And sometimes I think we could learn more from them
than they do from us

as we sit on our cushion bus
and ride to the sky

If we listened to kids
(and not to the adverts)
we might realise
where happiness lies

1 year 1 month

9.40 p.m.

Today I wrapped my lips around both of Little One's nostrils and sucked snot out of them. Like changing nappies and cleaning up sick, I do not find this OK because it is my child. I find it absolutely fucking gross. The result was good for her. I felt glad. I still feel sick thinking about it. Babies make me feel a bit sick quite a lot. Watching babies being spoonfed as the food gloop dribbles out of their mouths is another one that makes me a bit queasy. But this has definitely topped the list.

Deal With It

She had a cold.
Couldn't blow her nose
I was told: you just have to deal with it.

I wrapped my lips
Sucked the snot from it
Spat into the toilet, then vomited.

1 year 1 month

Teen Mums

She said
she tries to be yellow
but she's black

hiding all of the hurt
in her smiles and her handbag

Looked on as someone that's bad
as she pushes her kid in the pram

She said
that no one has any idea
what she's thinking or done or why she finds herself here

She said she spits out the looks and the tuts and the sneers
in the same grind of teeth as the panic and fear
that she feels.

I've just started a new workshop group with some young mums, writing poems about their experiences of motherhood and babies and, well, life in general. Today they were associating themselves with colours. I was chatting to a friend about the group. As soon as I started talking, she chipped in with her own story of 'teen mums'.

She was pretty scathing. Saw a group of girls – 'teen mums' – on the bus the other day. Described them as 'chatting to each other, just sitting texting, completely ignoring the babies'. 'Either way,' she said, rolling her eyes, 'they looked like they were having a pretty good day out, hanging about with their mates, going into town.' Then she added – 'I'm not being mean, I just feel sorry for the kids, you know.'

No, I do not fucking know. What I do know is that I work with a bloody lot of teenage mums and you don't, and I'm sick to shite of all this talk. What I also know is that right now she and I are also sitting chatting in town with our babies at the side of the table in prams.

It's not just other mums I hear this from. Every time I go into schools to do workshops, there is always at least one teenager, normally a pretty well-behaved, confident kid, one of the kids who's getting good marks, liked by the teachers, who writes about teenage mums – always a self-assuring poem about the problem of teenage mums, most often part of a creative description of the problems in their town or village.

The last school I went into, the 'teen mums strolling' figured in the same descriptive section of a poem about the town centre – 'rubbish bins overspilling, empty Coke bottles broken, teen mums strolling round with buggies'. Last week at a workshop, a fifteen-year-old lad described the 'sound of hate' as 'teen mums pushing prams', then proceeded to write a poem about how the teen mums in his school were terrible and why don't teenagers know how to use condoms and why don't they realise a baby is for life? Ah, it's that simple. Always that sodding simple. Well done you for being so damn honourable, you privileged young lad. Aside from that, in not one of these poems has a teen dad ever been mentioned.

So my friend finishes her description of these girls. And I say, well:

I text when I'm with my baby. It's pretty dull just being with a baby. They often don't chat a lot. I often text or call people while I'm pushing the pram round town.

I meet up with friends.

I don't constantly talk and interact with my child when I'm with her.

And neither does she. They're all assumptions we jump to when we see a group of mums who look as far from the white-linen middle-class-couple catalogue shot as you can get.

The more teen mums I meet, added to the more situations I find myself in with my child – being glared at, tutted at, or even just frowned at – the more I realise how horrible it is to be made to feel like a piece of shit for simply having a baby. I have constantly felt like I have done something wrong since having a big belly and then, even more, since pushing a pram. People seem to really hate mothers pushing prams. Teen mums especially. This week I drove to Manchester for a gig. Put on the radio to hear a 5 live chat show about 'gripes'. An older man was complaining about mums pushing prams as if 'they own the pavement'. 'Own the pavement' – that's exactly how I feel, yeah, when I'm trying to get round the shops before she needs to be changed, fed, comforted, to sleep. There is no chance to me that that man ever had to go to run errands and look after any kids at the same time. I wanted to smack that radio with my fist. Another blog last week put 'young mothers pushing prams while glued to their smart phones' into Room 101. Ahhh, that smug British sense of humour.

It really is amazing to me the way we treat teen mothers differently from other mothers. Don't get me wrong: older mums, working mums, stay-at-home mums – they're all good targets for society's finger. But with teenage mothers, it seems the immediate assumption is constantly that they are bad mothers, uninterested in the kids; doing it for the money, even. No idea of their backgrounds, wishes, how or why they had unprotected sex (as if none of us have ever done that, huh) got pregnant or, possibly most importantly, of their mothering skills.

And it is so two-faced.

If a group of our-age mums who met in an NCT class had walked past on the way to a coffee morning I'm sure that would have been seen as a *good* thing. Or just not seen as anything bad. Those mums are making support networks, they are taking their children out, getting fresh air, seeing new sights, making friends, drinking classy coffee. Everyone's a winner. Yet a group of teen mums do the same: meet with mum friends (often a lot harder to find for younger mums), chat (extremely important to have someone to relate to when you are in a minority like this), take their babies out (where they go is again trickier, as is the fact they feel more intimidated by the way people look at them with their babies), and the opinion is the exact opposite. For *those* mums, the chatting is equated to ignoring the babies, the meeting up with friends is equated to dossing around, having babies, skiving school and skanking off the state. And on a bus, eh. Mums taking their kids in a group on a bus to town, possibly in clothes that were not purchased in Next or White Stuff or Marks'n'Spencers. What a bunch of fucking slags.

But that's just it, I think. We might seem to be forward sexual thinkers in our British bubble, but since becoming a mum I really notice this shaming. Perhaps because, as a mother, people know you are (a) a female who has (b) had sex (c) without protection. I was twenty-six when I was pregnant and I still get a lot of comments – especially when my child is playing up. I've had people stop and stare at me, women on trains assuming the father has left (another bashing of younger people – the male variety), people shouting at me across the street or often simply telling me I'm 'too young' to have a child. Because at the end of the day, it's still deemed OK to shame a woman we think is too young to have had sex. Without knowing *anything* about them. As a culture, we totally obsess over young girls (and boys) bodies, sexing up fourteen-year-old models on catwalks and in catalogues, using images of open-legged waiting young females to sell every product under the sun, whilst still holding up the young virgin girl as the honourable high point of femininity. And well, of everyone, teen mums fuck that up. They're not sexy, young virgins posing on posters. Sexy would've been OK. But actual sex, well that's a sin. And yes, maybe in this free and loving country, unmarried teenage mums are no longer actually sent to asylums, or convents, or beaten or denied access to employment. But they are bloody well still shamed a great deal. And they know it. And it hurts them a lot.

Sometimes I just want to pretend; to make up a horribly tragic story; to look people who makes comments about me being 'too young' in the eye and say, 'Yes, I am fourteen, you're right. I was attacked and got pregnant. I had the baby and I'm now doing the best I can to raise this beautiful child.' Just so they shut the fuck up and realise they know nothing about my or any other parent's background. I know that wouldn't really be helpful, but I would like to see just one of the smug judgemental faces that these teenagers have faced in the last year crimson a little and walk away embarrassed.

The only thing I can do right now is just say 'No' in response to people's 'Do you know what I mean?' assumptions.

'No, I don't. Sounds like you saw a group of mums on a bus and totally judged them 'cos they were young, probably not very well off and in tracksuits.'

Even if it makes me unpopular. As for the school kids, I just have to keep questioning them whenever the holier-than-thou poems about pregnant girls and rubbish bins pop up – again, and again, and again.

It's a boring cog of conversation and I'm tired of it all. Those people who do not know any teen mums/teenagers/immigrants/other demonised members of society then go on a rampage about them, based on absolutely no factual information whatsoever. It always seems to be the people with the least actual experience of something who have the most prejudice. I guess that makes sense, though.

With class issues it seems that we're happier than ever to do that. Our radio does it, telly, films. Our very middle-class British satire programmes seem to love a bit of 'teen mum' bashing in a similar way to how they love a good dole queue, white van man or 'chav'.

Yuk. That's all, just yuk. I'm bored with it. 'Let he who is without sin' and all that.

A Perfect Tea Party

Last night I had a perfect cup of tea
passed to me by tiny hands and gasping eyes
who looked surprised
while I sat and sipped on air
stared as I declared:
'Delicious!'

She broke into fits of giggles
and slowly
dipped the teapot back into the bath
and filled the tiny plastic cup
as half spilled back on body parts

then held up with all her hands and heart
a bubble-loaded teacup
put it to her lips
and did her first fake sip

Glaring at me for support, unsure
she passed it back
I had another sip, sat up and said:
'Delicious!'
She clapped and
did the same.

One year old, proclaiming
'Mmmm!'
as she sipped on dirty bath water!

The first taste of make-believe
in a soapy bubbly cup of tea
a moustache of Matey
waiting patiently for the brain to turn it
into sweet and frothy cream

From then no looking back
no dream too grand
no need for toys now this is cracked
as toilet rolls are quickly snatched
telescopic paper packs
held to lips in speaker screams of
'Dadddeeeeee!'

Now every day I get a sweeter cup of tea
Brought to me by desert ladies
wrapped in towel shawls
climbing on my back
to hear my camel calls
she pats my back, claps
and lies back over it

My backbone is now a climbing frame
My stomach arched, a tunnel
My breath a tool
to blow out gales
hurricanes
and bubbles

and bubbles never fail

Throw the DVD, the TV, the nine-inch screen
the automatic speaking toys
plastic books that read themselves
the smell of cooking curry even
will not break her gaze
as bubbles float away
into the clouds
out of the window
across the path
into her bath
blown off covered palms

She laughs
and all the world's OK
'cos inside her mind's
a whole universe
of life

where dirty bathtime bubbles
are the best cup of tea you'll ever try.

11 p.m.

While I'm on baths . . .

I cannot count how many vouchers for baby products have now come through our door. Baby food, baby milk, baby products. Today's says: 'Best for baby. Best for you.' Shampoo. I remember the smell of the yellow baby shampoo from my days as a kid. And I get that shampoo that doesn't sting is helpful. I have a bottle of it in the bathroom. I've used it today. But they have so many products now and so much crap advertising sent through our door.

One ad claims:

'A warm bath with JOHNSON'S® Baby BEDTIME® Bath, a gentle massage with JOHNSON'S® Baby BEDTIME® Lotion, and a few minutes of quiet time. It's the clinically proven routine that leaves more time to dream.'

Then it says:

'Clinically proven to help baby fall asleep faster.'

I think: Faster than what? It doesn't say anywhere. But it matters what it's faster than, no? If it's scientifically proven to be faster, at least tell us faster than what!

Faster than having no routine at all?

Faster than a quick spray with a warmish shower and then bed?

Faster than giving your baby loads of boiled sweets, a glass of Coca-Cola and telling them to go to sleep whilst playing Giggs full blast?

Faster than what, Mr Johnson and Mr Johnson? Faster than *what*?

I look it up. It doesn't say anywhere on the website.

I know everyone's got their own routines: some of my mates bath their kids every night, some use lotions, some use creams because their baby's skin needs it. I use olive oil sometimes and shampoo her hair every two weeks. We're all different. But this marketing drives me nuts. Because it is making millions of pounds out of our babies when most of the products seem completely unnecessary. On top of that – I think the reason I get most annoyed – their claims take away the fact that me and Dee are doing all the bloody work here, not your goddamn clinically proven bottles of bath wash.

Argh. Faster than what? Stop with the science claims, people. Stop making money from babies, it's weird. We need that cash for when they grow up. I know it's our choice, so, sure, don't buy it. Sure, most of what we buy is unnecessary. I think it's just the number of leaflets I get. And the amount that they claim their products do. And how much I care I'm doing this right, so this stuff affects me more now. I feel way more vulnerable to it all. And they know that and obviously play on it a lot.

It's Us, Mr Johnson

Mr Johnson & Johnson's
I've a bit of a problem
with the things
that you're claiming you do

I don't doubt
your intentions are good (?!)
but I'll mention
a few of my worries to you

Your big purple bottle of bubble bath potion
claims it helps babies to sleep
and it's claims just like that that blur the truth of the fact
that the person working is *me*

'Cos it is night-time that helps
and bathtime that helps

and the warmth of the water around them that helps
and it's the routine that helps
and the stories that help
and the cosy towel hugging and swaying that helps

and all of that there, Mr Johnson, *we* do
It's got sod all to do with your bottle or you
You might argue your bath bubbles give a sleep smell
but any lavender scent would do that as well

So stop selling your products as some miracle cure
making claims like they're proven to help babies snore
using scientific words to make it sound truthful
'Formulas', 'professionals' and 'clinically proven'
'cos it blurs the truth of what us parents need
and your product alone does not help a child sleep.

And it seems like nothing. It's just a bottle. And I get that our Little One isn't the best sleeper. But it is a lot of money and waste for nothing.

This is the routine clinically proven to help baby sleep faster. Faster than a baby who has been washed in cold milk? Faster than a baby put to bed by an angry elephant? Faster than a baby put to bed in the middle of a drum'n'bass rave?

Step 1: A Warm Bath with JOHNSON'S® Baby BEDTIME® Bath

Help your little one let go of the day's excitement with a warm bath. JOHNSON'S® Baby BEDTIME® Bath is formulated with NATURALCALM® essences – a special blend of calming aromas. Held to our high standard of safety, this NO MORE TEARS® formula is as gentle to the eyes as pure water. For a bubblier start to your night-time routine, try JOHNSON'S® Baby BEDTIME® Bubble Bath & Wash!

Step 2: A Gentle Massage with JOHNSON'S Baby BEDTIME® Lotion

Follow the bath with a gentle massage. JOHNSON'S® Baby BEDTIME® Lotion is formulated with NATURALCALM® essences, a special blend that releases soothing aromas. Clinically shown to last all night long, this CLINICALLY PROVEN MILDNESS™ lotion formula is dermatologist-tested and hypoallergenic.

Step 3: Quietly Off to Sleep

After a warm bath and soothing massage, ease your little one off to sleep with quality quiet time together. Read a story, sing a lullaby or just quietly enjoy each other's warmth. Choose what works for you and your little one, but to ensure a good night's sleep, your quiet time shouldn't exceed twenty minutes.

So ... all good. But if I replaced each product with nothing at all, I think I'd get the same results. Only then, my baby's skin wouldn't be soaking up all the other ingredients in the bath product, which, as well as being formulated with NATURALCALM® essences, also include:

Water, PEG-80 Sorbitan Laurate, Cocamidopropyl Betaine, Sodium Laureth Sulfate, Sodium Lauroamphoacetate, Polysorbate 20, PEG-150 Distearate, Sodium Benzoate, Fragrance, Citric Acid, Sodium Hydroxide.

I am not a scientist and have no idea if these are good to be absorbed into a kid's bloodstream or not. All I know is that those ingredients are not shouted about as much on the website.

At the bottom of the page, the website says: 'OUR BABIES WILL INHERIT OUR PLANET™. Please Recycle.'

Or, perhaps, don't make believe we need to buy so many plastic products that do nothing, and save the plastic bottle being made in the first place? That'd help our babies inherit the planet.

No, no. It will help my Little One sleep faster and I'm told to 'use in a warm bath as part of your nightly routine'. Every night then? Use as much as they can possibly sell you. Every night, remember – at a time when you are willing to try absolutely everything to get some sleep. Inherit the planet my arse.

Yes, Mr Johnson and Mr Johnson, of course we should.

How much profit do you make again? How many different products do I need to make my baby sleep better? How many bottles of this stuff are floating around our babies' rivers?

And seriously – faster than what?

13 APRIL

1 year 1 month

9 p.m.

Sometimes I think Little One would be a bit freaked out if she knew how much I stand in her room in the dark and just stare at her face. I should probably stop. It's a bit odd. If I woke up and someone was staring at me in bed I'd call the police.

But I like watching her sleep. It reminds me that she is small and innocent and that it's ultimately up to us to protect her from everything right now.

Tiny

A few hours ago you were larger than life
lungs lined like a brass band
trumpeting vowel sounds
like practising drums
'Dadada' on repeat, until
'Ma'
'Mu'
'Mum'
'MUM!'

A few hours ago you were larger than life
my eyes vast, scanning knives
and other sharp objects
or buttons and coins
and all choke-hazard problems
on constant guard watch
as you run for the thrill
head far before legs
at that new-learner tilt,
where any moment your body is ready to
      tip
head heavy, mine too, as I sit on the ridge
ready to jump if you fall
at your beck and your call

A few hours ago you were larger than life
filling passers-by with your smiles
and then shyness
your eyes darting between the safety of my familiar
      legs
head clutched in both cheeks by my thighs
stumbling around through forests
and sunshine

A few hours ago you were larger than life
then you cried
in your cot
I go in
and you stop
with my hand
on your chest
once more

your breath rests
eyelids close
once again.

And I realise how tiny you are.

7

SUMMER
ONE YEAR THREE MONTHS
A MOVING KID

Play

Do You Remember?

Anyone's Anyone

Flesh

Terminator

20 MAY

1 year 2 months

7 p.m.

It is really warm today. The plum trees in the park are getting reading to burst into colour, covered in their sweet-scented blossom. I love this time of year. It is also a bit frustrating. There is a lot of talk (or advice!) of routine now and getting Little One to bed in her own bed at a similar time each evening. That she needs a pattern is fine – I understand it is a good idea. But it's now seven p.m. and she's asleep, which means I can't leave the flat. I can't go downstairs to the garden, even. I'm caged in. Caged in while it is a warm breezy evening outside, the perfect evening to sit out and have a cider or read a book in the summery dusk. I feel like I'm being taunted. The flat is quiet and calm and deliciously adult, but it is also hot and stuffy and has these things called windows reminding me how lovely the outside world is right now. Nope, I'll have to rethink this bedtime routine. Make it seasonal. Winter only. I don't want to be stuck inside from seven p.m. on a summer's night. No way. If she can sleep at Glastonbury, I'm sure she can sleep in the pushchair at the pub.

1 year 2 months

I am so damn tired. When I hear her morning shouts and check my phone and it is five a.m. or six a.m., I want to cry. Sob. Hysterically sob into my pillow. It's not morning yet but the sun is streaking through the tiny hole in the blinds. Blackout blinds, my arse. I know that this time last year I wasn't sleeping at all, but now that I have a taste of it every now and again, it's somehow worse. Go away, sun – I want winter back. The sleepy, dark mornings of winter. I hide under the warm covers and try to remember what a lie-in was like. I think I would sell my soul for a lie-in right now. Today is my day to get up, though, and Dee lies next to me blissfully snoring. She shouts again, I stumble out of bed mumbling something about just wanting to sleep and no one understanding how tired I am. I really feel like I am going to cry just because no one is listening to me moaning about this.

Then I get into her room, yawning till my eyes stream. She is standing, grabbing the cot, smiling, laughing and ready for the day, looking excitedly at dust fairies flying between the sun and the carpet, fluttering in that light stream beaming through the blind. She is in awe of the morning. Argh. How can I be annoyed with that? What a miserable cow I am. I smile back and pick her up and cry a bit. Out of tiredness and exhaustion and her smiling face. I get us ready to go to the park, washed, dressed, pram ready – and then realise it's only five-thirty a.m. Last week me and Dee and Little One went into town.

Wondered why the cafés were closed on a Saturday. Looked at Dee's watch. It was seven a.m.

Play

If only we could all play like children still play
I don't think we would be so depressed.
Picking myths out of daisy chains
Lips sipping whispering sounds into practising breaths

If only we could still think of objects as they do
without knowing their functional use
Eyes flickering awe at the kettle's first steam
and a boiling pan's cloud-shaded hue

If only we could feel the ground as they feel it
without thinking how messy we'd get
Lick the cold of a stone as our fingertips roam
into soil-laden mud-covered wet

If only we could still move like children still move
let notes jolt our limbs as they like
waving arms into spasms as laughter erupts
throwing tired chests down into night

If only we could wake up like children still wake
ready to take on the day
Six a.m. sunlight, already alive
impatiently waiting to play.

5 JUNE

1 year 3 months

2.15 p.m.

I went to visit Mum and Dad today. Bus, train, Tube, train. No lift at Paddington working. A guy carried the pram up the stairs for us and I felt my heart sing a little bit. I loved him at that moment. I have quite a love-and-hate relationship with strangers since having a child.

I took advantage of seeing mates back in Newbury – it's funny seeing friends without kids, which is most of my friends. It's lovely, but it's hard. I know it's more boring hanging out with me now. I can't concentrate on what they're talking about. They can see that. I apologise all the time:

Sorry, I just need to follow her.

Sorry, do you mind if I feed her?

Sorry, I've got to change her.

Sorry, what were you saying?

I met up with Caroline one day, only home mate who also has a kid. She asked me at one point what music I liked at the moment, if I was into any new groups. When I looked blank, she laughed. 'Just kidding, I can't even remember what clothes I like to wear any more.'

I thought about it. I couldn't either. I couldn't remember any new music or bands or fashion or anything. Anything I was into. What am I into? Who the fuck am I?! God, I love music.

Do You Remember?

Do you remember what it was like to feel awake?
Do you remember what it was like when your body didn't ache
and getting out of the house didn't take an hour and a half?
When you try not to cry but breathe in
When you are just out of the door and then just as you are
    leaving
your kid starts screaming and you have to go inside again
to change them?

Do you remember what it was like to have a shower or a bath
uninterrupted
without little faces peering over the bathtub
begging to get in?

Do you remember what it was like to feel comfortable in your
    own skin?
Before looking at your body consisted of memories of before?
Do you remember the times you could admit to being bored
(without feeling guilty?)
Before speaking secretly to other parents about craving adult
    talk?
About how slow your toddler walks?
Do you remember what it was like to talk to people your own
    age?
To engage in conversation that made your brain feel tight again?
Do you remember your body before it made and fed and raised
    a life?

Do you remember what things you like?
Do you remember your own hobbies?

Or what it's like to have some space to think?
Or take a bath or drink a tea while it still steams
To have a wee in peace?

Do you remember the days before you knew how this love really
    felt?
Love so strong some days you feel you've sacrificed yourself for
    them?
Body, heart and mind
and then some more?

And some days you long to crawl
body dragged across the floor
roll over on your back
and stare up at the ceiling
pleading
'Please
PLEASE!
Please just leave me here
to lie down
to close my eyes
and sleep some time'

but no one's there to hear your cries!

so you carry on instead
and do not really mind
as long as that little sunshine of a child
smiles from time to time.

3 p.m.

I feel like phoning all my friends and telling them to stay in bed. Spend the day listening to music. Reading books. Go and watch as many bands as you can afford to. Watch them on YouTube if you can't. Savour themselves and their own company right now if they are even considering having children at some point. Don't feel bad about it. Just chill. Laze. Relax.

But I know it won't make any difference. Until you don't have time to yourself very much, I guess you don't know how much you appreciate it. Today was appreciated. I can't believe I used to do this all the time and didn't appreciate the beauty of being alone to chill out. It is a beautiful, sacred thing. My third spiritual experience in life. The second was watching pear juice drip from my child's face. The first was birth. This one is less traumatic.

Anyone's Anyone

Today I don't have to be anyone's anyone
Baby and boyfriend both away
I've got seven hours just to lie by myself
Hot tea. A book. A whole day.

Today I don't have to be anyone's anyone
My thigh dimples can sigh and relax
No one to look or squeeze them at all
No thoughts about cycling or wax.

My hair can stay messy, my toenails uncut
My feet can breathe out, free of socks, covered up
My eyes can stay narrow, mascara away
'Cos it is me and my bed and a book for the day.

My pyjamas with stains will stay on my skin
And my stomach untensed can stop breathing in
My breasts can chill out for a day without grabs
Whether baby for milk or a frustrated dad.

I have had two straight years as a mother and mum
And now seven hours to be nothing for no one
I've had seven years as a girlfriend and lover
And now seven hours to be none of the other.

I can pick my nose, bite my toes, leave my cup on the floor
I can go to the toilet and not close the door
I can shower without any eyes wanting looks
I can nibble without anyone needing cooks.

'Cos today I don't have to be anyone's anyone
Seven hours completely for me
So when boyfriend and baby come back from their day
I'll be mum and I'll be lover
and pleased.

7 JUNE

1 year 3 months

Flesh

Savour the feeling, Hollie, because in a second it'll be gone
Her tiny fingertips won't search your chest for very long
So close your eyes and try to remember each press
The pad of each tap on your flesh.

1 year 5 months

Little One has been walking and exploring all summer. I am a nervous wreck! She is trying to eat soil, stones, leaves, dirt. I am so tired right in the centre of my brain. I feel like I am using parts of my brain I never knew I had before. Mushy mummy baby brain is definitely a joke. I am using five times my brain capacity now. She is walking faster and faster each day and my eyes cannot move from her sight. The minute I look for something or do something, I come back and she'll have a new dangerous object about to enter her mouth or a table corner in her toddling line. My brain, the concentration segment (if there is one), is being pushed to the max. I am Terminator.

Terminator

My world feels like a GCSE physics test –
Page ten, a pencilled kitchen sketch
where open plugs and scissors rest
left for you to take a red pen to
and circle all five hazards you can see

It was easy at the time –
broken wires near water

open plugs
scissors sticking up
people slipping up
on scattered nuts across the floor

They were obvious back then
in the GCSE physics test
but now there's no set score
and no one says how many you've to find
and now it's not a test
but I am more desperate now than ever
to get them all correct

My pen clutched in sweaty palm
searching hard for new alarms
for sharp things left on floors
or open plugs

The world is one big hazards test
since I became a mum.

and I am circling constantly
desperate to see them all
my normal sight replaced
by this widened-vision panic call

and I was told about the other things
waking nights and smiles and crying
but I never thought I'd worry quite so much
about a baby dying
after she was safely born and fed

and in my head
I feel a bit like Terminator One
with death-defying goggles on
and every time I spy a plug or wire
the infra beam starts going off –
Information sheets rolling down
flashing lists in both my eyes
of all the ways in which these hazards
might mean that
my baby dies

And it all just sounds so morbid
and now I'm drawing circles round the sky
red pen strewn across her walkways
every minute by her side

Just circling these hazards
I am circling them once again
and circling them fifty times
to make sure they're not drawn again

and when you say I've lost my memory
my mind seems slightly scattered
it's 'cos I'm trying to save a baby's life
from things that haven't happened
from things that I imagine
from things that could go wrong
and I'm worried sick every day
that my hazard beams will not be strong
        enough
tomorrow

As I circle stuff
like boiling pans
and table edges
cars and tree tops
pavements
pen lids
and when she sleeps I still can't stop
I circle
bedclothes
pillows
pyjama buttons
falling shelves
light bulbs burning
bolt upright every time she's turning
in her sleep

Every time she snores or breathes

And each day reaps a thousand more
each page of life a thousand sores
each thousand minutes more amazing
each day she grows my pen goes crazy
repeating desperately to see she's understood
when I say

Stop. Wait. Look both ways. Think it through.

I gave her a red pen last week
and a circle was the first thing that she drew.

And no one told me this would happen
when I chose to raise a child

that my mind would readjust
and an inbuilt beam replace my eyes
that my life would be a constant test
of circling the hazards
and that I'd worry every second
about the ones that I can't manage
or control

and now she's walking on her own
and she knows what not to touch
and she points to scissors, shows me
and shakes her head at open plugs

and my life is like a hazards test
the circles getting slightly smaller
my pen now helping hers to draw
and my own – to reinforce her.

1 year 5 months

I really want to quit my job. Not poetry, the day job. I don't think I can carry on with everything. I'm getting more gigs and workshops than I could've ever imagined and combining two jobs with gigs and parenting is turning me into a zombie. Last week one of the other poets who had booked me asked me to write a new poem for the gig I was doing that week. He didn't say that at first, then just asked out of the blue. He gave me two days' notice. I kind of snapped – 'No I can't sorry – are you kidding?'

'Come on, Hollie,' he said, 'it's a paid gig and you've got two days.'

I repeated, 'No, I can't, sorry.'

I was polite. He was really pissed off. So many people I work with seem to have no rent, no kids, no day job. No idea how busy every minute of my life is. And I can't write poems on demand, anyhow, I never have. I write when they come into my head. Most of the time nowadays I lose them because I can't stop and write as I'm running across the park shouting 'Watch out for the stinging nettles!' or 'Mind the swings!'

I got a call from the BBC last week to go on the radio, 'Today at two p.m.' Nice notice! I know this is 'how the industry works' but it is impossible for a working parent. Or working anyone. And annoying, because it was such an opportunity.

But last night's gig has made me think seriously about quitting my job. Kate Tempest asked me to do a support set at her book launch. Kate Tempest at the Old Vic in London. She is a genius and I have been excited about this gig for months. Completely stoked to be asked. Dee and Little One came to London with me and played in the dressing room. I fed her before I went on stage. The theatre was full. I read out three poems. Everyone listened and clapped and hopefully liked them. Three hundred people listening to my poems. It was daunting and made me feel sick but so damn grateful. Kate did her set and it was bloody brilliant. Little One ran on the stage by accident then fell asleep in the dressing room. So did Dee. I mean, he fell asleep. He didn't run onto the stage. We got home a bit past midnight.

The next morning I got up at six a.m. and cycled to work at eight, still buzzing from the night before. The trustees were having their meeting and for the first time I was invited. I've been managing the education section in the office for nearly a year and finally they wanted to 'make me part of the meetings, show I'm a valued team member'. So they all come in and I feel a bit sick as I always do when they come in. They smile at me and are polite as ever and tell me what tea they want. I ask the last trustee if he'd like a coffee or tea and he says, 'Uh, water?'

I go to the kitchen to make the teas, at which point the trustees shut the office door on me and start the meeting. I stand in the tiny tea room boiling the kettle realising that they've forgotten that they invited me to the meeting. Forgotten, and also do not know or probably give a damn that that invitation was a really big deal for me. I consider walking home. I'm embarrassed. Instead I make the tea and open the door, my face bright red with awkwardness. 'Oh, sorry Hollie,' they laugh, 'we forgot about you.'

Life is so surreal. Last night I read a poem to three hundred people about how proud I was to be a woman and a mum. I then watched the most amazing poet spill her heart out to them all. Now I'm back to making tea and having the door shut in my face. If I'm going to give up something, this should be it. I just don't know if I can afford to give up a steady salary right now. And I don't hate the job, I love the team. I love the work. Just not the trustee meetings. Or making tea for people who seem to think that's all I'm good for. Or the fact that the job relies on funding and I could be made redundant at any time.

I try to focus on last night's gig, on Kate's words, on the audience's laughter, as I sit smiling at a group of 'superiors' telling me for the fiftieth time that they would prefer me not to use Helvetica in the next project brochure. Give a shit. Drink your fucking tea, I think. Be happy I like fonts so much.

8

AUTUMN
ONE YEAR SIX MONTHS
GOING AWAY

Hotel Sheets

Computers Cannot Kiss

Heavy Hands

1 SEPTEMBER

1 year 5 months

7 p.m.

It's quite nice when the small things give me a rush of feeling like I've achieved something massive. The plums are ripe in the park, so every night after dinner now I go and eat them with Little One, for pudding. She's like a human grabber tool. Last night I had to scale a pretty high tree to get the ones I wanted. I left Little One on the ground, on a path with fairly high stinging nettles either side and said 'Stay.' And she did. I got the plums. We ate them. She did not get stung. Little things. My daughter stood still when I asked. And I feel like I am a fucking don!

The plums are juicy right now. I got a Google map today of local fruit trees and now have a pretty good route into work on the bike which takes me past three types of plums, as well as figs, pears, apples and wild city strawberries.

I think my parents forced into me a love of free things, and I currently live in a place where the local park has enough fruit to save me three months' worth of shopping for it. It's immense. Sometimes I find it boring living in a small village, but when the fruit is free, it pretty much makes up for any of those feelings. Now I have a kid, the calmness of this place is lovely. And the free food makes my heart sing.

Whenever my gran got the train from Scotland to England to visit, she would come bounding into the house laden with sugar sachets from the train, her excuse being that they would've thrown them out otherwise "cos they were on my saucer already'. Thing is, they were only on her saucer in the first place because she would order eight sugars so that she'd have the excuse to nick them after she didn't use them.

My gran also seems to have handed down a summer-fête-free-scones-and-tea radar to my dad, who almost crashes the car whenever we're in Scotland and he sees some sort of fête or parade. 'We'll just take a look,' he says, hunting out the 20p cakes: 'Homemade, Hollie – let's go.' My gran is better at it still, and is a vital guide on trips to Loch Lomond, knowing exactly which shops give out free tablet tasters and Tunnock's, as well as what weeks in the year the local churches and halls have free tea and biscuits.

So the free fruit is good. Even more so now, because it is also the way I'm weaning Little One off the last night-time feed. Instead of feeding her breastmilk before bed, we go to the park and gorge on plums – and figs – free, and I pretend I live in a stately home with an orchard.

I think, as well as stuffing her, it also distracts me from the fact that I'm pretty sad about the end of night feeding. It's the second-to-last feed left and I'm stopping it. No more. Never, ever again. I will never get this back. Never feed her at night and watch her slowly drift off, drunk, into the land of nod. These new freedoms are weird. On the one hand I want to run around jumping for joy – I can go out! I can go to gigs by myself without Dee or my mum having to haul their arses around the country just because this night-time feed clashes with gig-set times. I can stop feeling guilty that I didn't seem to be able to pump milk at all.

On the other hand, though, every time I put her into her cot at the moment, I want to break down in tears and curse the plums and pray they have enough nutrients and goodness to make up for the contin-uous decline in her system of my antibody miracle juice. I'm petrified now that the food I give her won't be good enough. I don't even know why I'm stopping these feeds. Mainly, I think, because of the pressure from everyone around me who now thinks it's 'getting weird'. Not Dee. He has been the most supportive partner I could've imagined. But a lot of others. I feel I'm caving into pressure the same way I did when I went for a bikini wax and put the paper pants on the wrong way round, wondering why they were sticking up my fanny so much. My cousin Tracy thought it was funny anyway. That was the one and only time I went for one. Fuck that pain, I'll just buy bigger pants. And fuck you plums, even if you are free and bloody delicious.

I also, selfishly, hate the fact that Little One doesn't have to come to gigs any more. I know my mum and Dee will be well happy, but it was really nice having them there. Having Dee and Little One share all those trips, pegging it down the M4, feeding backstage and hoping my boob wasn't leaking milk onto my top in front of the audience. It's nice not to go to gigs alone, because sometimes it's a bit like going on a night out by yourself. Sit on your own awkwardly, go on stage, read some poems, then sit on your own awkwardly some more. I sometimes hide in toilets in the breaks 'cos I don't know what to do or to say to people. I didn't have to do that with the family gig trips. I'll have to hide in toilets in gig breaks again now. Damn!

This shit is so emotional. Freeing and petrifying. If I wanted another child, maybe it'd be different. But I don't. Having one child is beautiful, even if people feel the need to tell me she will be lonely and spoilt. But I'll do my hardest to make neither of those the case. Just one. So whenever any experience stops now, it makes me think – *You will never have that experience ever again*. Never. I will never feed her into sleep ever again.

I watch her sleeping, eat a plum, and sob. Sob like I have never sobbed before. Dee comes in and we sit in the dark hugging it out. I'm free. Great, I'm free.

1 year 6 months

9 p.m.

I am sitting on the bench in the park in the village with a screw-top bottle of rosé wine pressed to my lips. Little One is sleeping (I hope) at home two minutes away. Our friend is babysitting.

She thinks I'm out at a gig but I'm not. Instead I am in tears on my own in the dark with a bottle of wine on a bench, hoping no one I know walks past and asks me what the hell I'm doing. I'm not sure I've cried this much since the boy I fancied through school refused to snog me at a party and I drank half a bottle of wine and sobbed until my mascara made my cheeks look like a swollen red-blotched black-watercolour painting. I sat in the toilet at the party while my drunk friends tried to console me. The next Monday at school I felt like a twat and I'm sure I will feel the same tomorrow. This is not a big deal, I know that. I have a lovely family and a healthy child and I feel guilty with every tear that wets my cheeks, but I can't stop. I am officially feeling sorry for myself.

There was a poetry night tonight I wanted to go to. At the local theatre. A one-hour show I've always wanted to see by a guy called Polarbear. I can't get out very easily, I have been feeding a child for nearly two years and now have no more night-time feeds and I was so excited Polarbear's show was coming to Cambridge Junction. I can go to the show! I can actually go to the show! It's only £5 as well. Score. So, as you have to do now as a mum, I asked permission to go. I found a sitter, as Dee's away working. I got Little One ready for bed on time – in bed, on time – all done perfectly. I got ready. Put mascara and my orangey-pink lipstick on – the in-colour right now. First time in ages I've been so made up. Got ready, on time, put on a pair of earrings, which means I must be doing something exciting because I can only wear those when there's no small fingers to pull them through my skin and rip my ears right out of my head. I did everything perfectly, everything ready. I sat watching the clock, excited. Excited to be going out by myself. No kid. No mum role. The show is only one hour long. I planned to get there half an hour early, have a drink by myself. Sit, quietly, as an adult, in a theatre. Not a soft play centre or a park or a toddler group. In an actual adult theatre. Go and see the show and come back. I have bigged this day up in my head for the last two weeks. I AM GOING OUT SOMEWHERE! I WILL WEAR EARRINGS! I WILL DRINK A GLASS OF WINE! I HAVE NEW LIPSTICK!

Seven o'clock came. No one showed. I'm ready, sat with my coat on and bag over my shoulders, legs twitching, ticket in the side pocket, fiver in my purse. She'll be here at seven p.m.

Seven-fifteen comes. Still waiting. Start feeling a bit stupid. I shouldn't have put so much into this evening. It's just that I haven't done something for myself, by myself, for a long, long time.

Seven forty-five. Lipstick is licked off. I reapply it. I've now missed my chance at a drink first. But no bother, bit disappointed, but it's just a drink.

Seven-fifty, she's here. 'Sorry I'm late, have a great time!' 'Thanks so much,' I say. And I *am* thankful, but I just wish she wasn't forty-five minutes late. I only had two hours tonight anyway, but it was two hours for me. Now it's down to one hour and a quarter. Better than nothing still. I pick up my bag, kiss Little One in the cot, race out of the door. I phone the theatre on the way.

'I've got a ticket for Polarbear's eight p.m. show. I'm running ten minutes late. Can I come in late if I'm really quiet?'

'Sorry. No latecomers I'm afraid, the show's only an hour long you know?'

Yes. I know. I was ready. But no one else was. No one understands.

I offer to crawl in under the chairs as quiet as a baby mouse on a feather duvet.

'I'm afraid you can't – really sorry.'

I am now in my car, dressed up and made up, I've missed my drink and on the way to see a show I can't get into. I look at my bag on the passenger seat with a fiver for a glass of wine inside. I imagine going home and saying: 'I missed the show, don't worry about babysitting ever again as I will never be able to go out ever again and I now realise that. I was being a fool to try.' Over the top, for sure. But I cry a little about the idea of going home early. I know it's not a big thing. I know it's not, I really do. But it's just that no one seems to understand what a big thing it was to me to just go somewhere alone and do something I like doing. Even when it's still kind of for work.

I turn the car around and pull into One Stop, wiping my mascara smudges a bit. I buy a bottle of screw-top rosé wine and park the car at the end of our road. I look for a place to sit and feel like a teenager again scouting for bridges or benches to get drunk with friends after managing to get underage-served at a local shop. I think that was a One Stop too. I didn't ever get served. I looked twelve till I was about twenty. Kathryn or Hannah did. But I was part of the team.

I sit on the bench. In the dark. On my own. Feel like a complete fool and cry, sipping from the bottle, thinking of those days with my friends, passing it between us. I refuse to go home until my hour is done, partly because I don't want to, partly because I'm embarrassed. Feeling stupid for getting my hopes up. Feeling guilty for wanting to be on my own. Or away from my mum role. Away from that gorgeous little child. I imagine her sleeping, oblivious to her stupid mum with her new lipstick on and I cry some more and take a few more slugs.

It's nine p.m. The show has finished. I walk to the car and check my face in the mirror. I wipe my mascara again and redo my make-up, attempting to look like I did when I left. I wait five minutes for my cheeks to be less red and chuck the leftovers of the wine bottle in the bin.

I get into the flat.

'Thanks,' I say. 'Was she OK?'

'Yes, she never moved an inch. How was the show?'

'Good,' I say. I'm sure it was good. Polarbear's shows are always good.

I thank her again and she leaves. I go into Little One's room and give her a kiss and an apology for being such a fool. I sit on the sofa and watch repeats of *A Place in the Sun*, feeling like a spoilt cry-baby and vowing not to bother trying to go out again. I think about my friends from school. I wish they lived closer. I miss my friends a lot.

2 OCTOBER

1 year 6 months

10 a.m.

Everything about being a mum makes me feel guilty. I woke up this morning feeling guilty. I have been away one night. One night. I feel free and guilty. Free, free and guilty! Guilty that I love the feel of these hotel covers and the creased pillow and the sleep. Guilty that before I went, my friend told me: 'You won't cope. I couldn't take being away from my child for one night, I had to come home.'

But ... I don't feel like that at all. I think I like it. I think if anything I want to go away more. To give Dee some time, proper time, day-and-night-and-day-again time when I'm not there at all. It's important. Because if I'm there, she wants me more. I feel like I'm only saying that so I can bugger off again, but I'm not. I didn't really think about it before. That he's never had a day and then a night and then a day again with her. It is important. And it feels bloody good to get some proper sleep. And the stiff white sheets! Fucking aida, the stiff white sheets! Someone told me I'd wake up all night anyway because that was my routine now. No chance. As long as I know she's OK, I can sleep. And she's OK with her dad. I slept like a bloody log. I feel guilty that I slept like a log. And the lie-in. Words cannot describe that.

Hotel Sheets

First night away from my little one
I couldn't fall asleep at first
Checking photos on my phone
Kissing screens in lovesick moans
My eyes start drooping into sleep
I think of you now out of reach
And force my head to see the fact
That you and dad are all enwrapped
Around each other, safe as two
And me away is good for you
And for the first time in two years
I slept for seven hours clear
My eyelids opened without pain
And a little rest back in my brain
No morning moanings to and fro
I'll go, Dee
No it's all right
I'll go
No little hand to poke my face
Begging me to start the day
But what I'll say despite the lack
Despite the morning full of gaps
I had a fucking good night's sleep
But you weren't there to wake me
I had a lovely full night's sleep
But you weren't there to wake me
I didn't miss the five-up start
But I missed who makes that happen
I missed the man asleep with me
Giggling with tired glee

As you climb up, awake all three
I missed your smile
I miss your pleas
But I had a fucking good night's sleep!
In crisp white sheets

I had a good night's sleep.

1 year 6 months

5 p.m.

Computers Cannot Kiss

I can hear children laughing
I miss my little kid

I read her a story on Skype last night
but computers cannot kiss

I put my lips up to the screen but
I really miss her skin.

I read a story over Skype
last night
but computers cannot kiss.

4 OCTOBER

Nearly 1 year 6 months

Going away has really made me think. Mainly because I loved it. I missed them. But. I. Loved. It. I loved being on my own. I loved the fact that I was far enough away that I couldn't worry about Little One. There was no need to prick up my ears all night because I couldn't hear her. It was a blessed feeling and I realise now that I have not slept properly at all since the very day she was born. I am always on alert, always, even in my sleep. The slightest noise and I am awake.

Funny thing is, when I got back, Dee said he woke up loads more than normal. He doesn't normally wake that much. It used to piss me off. I'd be woken up at the smallest fucking noise and he'd be lying there sleeping, snoring, like nothing was happening and I'd want to punch his lights out. A little bit. Mainly, though, I'd be pleased that he wasn't as tired as me when the morning alarm came on. There's no point us both being awake and then exhausted. I used to think it was a biological difference between men and women. Now I think it's just because he's relaxed knowing I'm there, but will definitely wake up a lot more when I'm not.

Being away also made me realise that it is a good thing to do. It is a great thing to have a partner I can go away from with no worries. Everything that has led up to this has been worth it: taking turns doing bedtimes, mornings, both going to the toddler group. The more you share, the more you're going to be able to 'get away' later. There are so many people who don't have that. Not just single parents, but – well, mainly – mums who don't leave the kid with their partner because he doesn't have experience looking after them on his own. Sometimes I think it's the man who's being a lazy ass, sometimes I think it's the woman who's being overly worried and maybe not letting the guy spend the time with the child that he'd need so as to become confident on his own.

Sometimes I think it's just way more complicated than either theory. My dad still won't have Little One by himself. Lots of men I know won't look after children alone, not even their own kids. Whoever's to blame for that situation, I'm glad I'm not in it. Knowing that Little One is fine, Dee is fine, everything is fine if I go away for a night, do a gig and sleep cosily in a crisp, clean, beautiful, soft, perfect bed all to myself – well, it's bliss.

I feel like I can spiral up or down from here. I'm going up. I need this to always be OK. It is liberating to know I'm not needed twenty-four hours a day, every day. That I'm really, honestly, not. Like, it really is OK if I go somewhere else sometimes. I'm trying to convince myself. No one is going to explode. Not even the kid. I think Dee knew that a while back. My guilt just stopped me from fully believing him.

10 OCTOBER

1 year 7 months

1 a.m.

Yesterday was the most surreal day I've ever had. Dreich, bleak, miserable, deflating. I came back from what was meant to be five days working on a show at Battersea Arts Centre after just one day, because Little One is ill. She was being sick all over the studio room I was working in, so we decided best not stay! Dee had come with me to London for five days to look after her, but the idea of spending all that time in a theatre with an ill child is not a good one. Not fair on either of them. So we left to drive home. Disappointing, because that theatre is possibly the most parent-friendly amazing place I have ever worked in. After all the opportunities I have had to miss in this artsy poetry planet solely because I could not work it into parenthood, finding Battersea Arts Centre felt like the scene in *The Goonies* where they finally come across the pirate ship with One-Eyed Willy. I think that was his name. What a cracking film. Not only have they got an indoor play area café for kids here, so I can actually work as my daughter runs riot in an enclosed heaven, they have bedrooms we can stay in, producers to help and rooms for work. It is a bloody dream.

Anyway, we had to leave. Driving back, and just by Bow, East London, the car packed up. Little One's sick by the roadside, Dee phoned the mechanic. On the phone, he opened the bonnet and hub cap. I have no idea why he was told to do this but he screamed, clutching his fist and the top of his head, burnt from the boiling steam. Thank fuck it did not hit his eyes, nose or mouth and that it wasn't worse. I called the ambulance and the AA as I sprinted to the nearest shops to hunt for a bag of ice, frozen peas, anything, Little One clinging to my back, stopping whenever she needed to throw up. We got back and the ambulance was there giving Dee a cold pack and bandaging his forehead and fist. Bless the NHS. He looked like he'd been in a bad fight. I get my breathe back. Little One sits on the pavement playing with a stick.

The AA van came, took us as far as the A406 McDonald's before they realise they've brought the wrong car to tow us back home. They tell us it's going to be a two-hour wait. OK, whatever, we feel lucky to have an AA at all. So we went into McDonald's. At nine p.m. With Dee all wrapped up like a fight victim. I ordered some chips, as we hadn't eaten for hours. Little One suddenly vomited on the counter, all over it, and I ran to the toilet with her, apologising to the staff and asking for tissues and mop. I smelled like vomit and we looked like the grimmest family ever, taking a beaten-up bloke and a vomiting toddler out to eat chips at nine p.m. on a dark, cold night. At that point I make a pact never to judge anyone ever again. The McDonald's staff are the most helpful people I have ever met in my life. I want to kiss them all. But I smell of vomit and baby tears so decide not to.

The AA van came to get us at eleven p.m., driven by a middle-aged man who was about to get British citizenship after moving to the UK eight years ago. He's very friendly until he starts telling us that the only bad thing about the UK is that 'we're too open to foreigners'.

'You need to have tighter immigration controls,' he said, then started talking about a rich 'Indian' (British) man he picked up once who had bought a Mercedes car with child benefits. Uh huh. Sure thing. We talked about it, but it's a pretty hard situation, getting into an argument with someone who's your only way of getting you and your sick child home.

Dee had a gig that started at midnight and he insisted on going to it. The AA man dropped him off at the nightclub on the way. As soon as Dee got out of the car, the driver turned round to me, at midnight, on my own in the back of a huge AA truck clutching an ill, sleeping toddler and says:

'Did you always want a black man, then?'

Perfect end to a perfect day. I love this question. Haven't been asked it in a while. I smiled. 'No.'

He takes it the wrong way.

'So, why didn't you go for a white man if you didn't want a black man?'

It was far too late for this, I was far too tired to be stuck in an AA van with a racist driver who I cannot argue with because I am on my own with a baby and he is massive and I am small and weak and he is my only way home.

'No, I didn't. I wanted him because we got on. We got on because we both write. We met and started reading our stories to each other. That was why we started dating. Because we got on with each other.'

Nah, he doesn't care.

'How do your family feel about you dating a black man?'

'They are just happy he's not English,' I say. 'My family is Scottish. They hate the English.'

'Oh, OK,' he says.

'I'm joking,' I say. 'He *is* English. And my family like him.'

He kept on at me all the way home. Interesting how he didn't start this conversation with Dee in the actual vehicle. Weak.

He mentioned our 'confused' kid. That's enough.

I will write to the AA tomorrow. Right now, I just want a cup of tea, my arms free and a shower.

Heavy Hands

Did you always go for black men?
Did you always want a black man?
Did you always go for dark skin?

No I didn't.
I went for *him*.

One man. With a name
whose smile made my day
as we chatted about his teaching job
and I crossed the road in football socks
and muddy knees
and he waved to me
and the talk flowed out so easily
and we realised
that we both loved to write
and that we both wrote in A4 notebooks
and stayed up scribbling late at night.

My last boyfriends were white
No one asked me why I liked their skin
if I always dated men
who looked a little bit like them

So,
Did you always go for white men?
Did you always like a white man?
Did you always want a light man?
No one ever asked me that.

And when my belly swelled in love
and I was vomiting for six full months
and he was like a goddamn angel
a halo cap he tipped my way
who refilled ice trays desperately
and fed my cravings best he could
and sang songs to the kicking limbs
and the baby healthy heard within
still,
you asked about his skin

Not,
Did you always want a kind man?
Did you always want the kind of man
who reads stories to his unborn kid
and dances in elfin long johns
just to cheer me up while I am sick
and helps to hold my hair back?

Just,
Did you always like them black?
Just,
You always liked them black!

And when the baby came, a new cry
Did you always want a mixed child?
A caramel-skinned curly-haired child?
they said
seriously.
not a healthy child, or a happy child
or a child-whose-dad-changes-more-nappies child
than I do

as different skin tones open flat-pack boxes
thick to push you into

Personalities left aside as people ask
– exoticising
– interested
– why I hooked up with that black guy?
as if that is the *only* choice I made
and why I think he chose a white girl
as my mind and brain are all erased
and what a lovely tone our child is
now we mixed between our race

A tone, I'm told, is
'just right'
'Not too dark, not too light'

Not too light like me, you mean!
Transparent Scottish tones and freckly?
Not too dark like him, you mean!
The kind of brown he's got
that makes him picked on by police
and stopped at customs
every time we leave to go away?

Like colour is a fashion taste
as if we both care more about the tone
of our newborn baby's face
than her health
and love
and heart rate

It's a hard race to win
and some days I just say yes,
I have been looking
for a brown-skinned man to date
since I was interested in sex
and I spent all my teenage life
studied hard and worked all night
just to try to find a black man
who wants a white chick in his life

So I sigh and walk away
on a path where pigment paves the way
let the night air cool my face
as I watch the A A man escape

and the next day
I watch their lovely faces
dad and daughter clowning round
as they gaze at one another
as she stumbles up another branch
of the tree we always climb
and he watches like a nervous wreck
trying to hide his mind
petrified of the step her foot might miss
ready to catch her with a kiss

So I'll tell you my real answer, sir –
I always wanted to date someone like this

I always wanted to date someone
who'd hold out heavy hands
below tree branches
just in case their daughter slipped.

9

WINTER
ONE YEAR EIGHT MONTHS
AUSTRALIA AND GRANDMAS

1 NOVEMBER

1 year 7 months

4 a.m. (Sydney time)

I would like to kiss the feet of whoever has encouraged me to continue breastfeeding until now. Dee. Dee's gran – Ionie. Mum. Little One. Parent friends at toddler group.

Thank you.

Thank you.

Thank you.

I love you.

The flight to Australia was booked over a year ago and when I said that to one of the mums at toddler group, she said, 'Well, just carry on feeding her if you can. Breastfeeding on a long-haul flight is a good trick.'

How right she was.

The funny thing is, I have also been using this flight as an excuse to carry on feeding, because I feel embarrassed about it again. It's one thing to feed a baby, but as soon as Little One hit six months old, the pressure to stop started to mount up.

Why are you still feeding if she can eat food?

Why are you still feeding if she can talk?

Why . . . ?

Why . . . ?

Nosy bastards.

Why . . . ?

The first in the list was the most common question. *But if she can eat food . . . why?* That, and people assuming I was still only giving her breastmilk when she was one and a half. As a society, we really know so little about this stuff, it's unreal. But we still feel pretty confident giving advice – or, more like, judging – about things we know fuck all about.

So for the last six months I have been feeding her at five a.m., meaning I get to lie in for an extra two hours. But I stopped feeding in public a while ago. And I stopped being honest about the feeding – saying things like 'Oh, I'm just feeding her till we go to Australia, 'cos it's helpful for the flight.' The pressure to stop was so strong. I just don't see why people give such a shit.

Why are you still feeding her?
Why not use follow-on milk now?
It's a bit weird now she can talk?
So does she walk up and ask . . . you know?!
Oh my God, does she say 'bitty'?
Don't you find it strange?

I'll be honest. Yes, I do find it fucking strange! I do find it strange feeding a kid who can talk. And walk. But I think the only reason I find it strange is because you all keep looking at me weirdly and *telling* me it's strange. And it makes me feel like absolute shit. Even when it's no problem. Even if I did stop feeding her, I'd have to start spending money on powdered milk and give her that instead, when I could just carry on feeding her my own goddamn free milk.

I really want to move people's attention away from this subject completely, because I don't understand what our fucking problem is with this. Judge something else, not this, which does no harm to anyone and doesn't affect you in the slightest. I am not making a point. I am not anti-bottle. I do not get a kick out of it. I am just feeding my kid and saving a lot of money, 'cos I can and 'cos it's recommended and 'cos I have no trouble doing it. No trouble except feeling fucking weird about it now.

I want to take people's cheeks between my palms when they go on about this or make wee quips or jokes, and say 'Perhaps try to focus on actual problems.'

Like, if you ask:

Why are you still feeding, Hollie? I'll say: 'Why are kids being bullied so badly they kill themselves? Why not worry about that.'

Is it not a bit weird now, Hollie? I'll say: 'Not as weird as the fact that most of the world's wealth is owned by a tiny minority, while half the world starve. Why not worry about that.'

When are you gonna stop then? I'll say: 'Hate crimes, I wonder when they'll stop.'

Some actual things to worry about. Breastfeeding a toddler, not one of them. Stop judging. Stop bothering yourselves about a kid being fed. It's a waste of my and your energy.

I was worried about the flight purely because it would be in public, and my kid can talk, and because that fact combined with the fact of breastfeeding, in this fucked-up world, is frowned upon. But it was fine. It was magic. It was like having a breast-shaped wand that got rid of hunger, earache, nerves, sleep deprivation and crying with one flash of a perky nipple.

The flight went a bit like this:

Take off –

Little One's ears popped

Boob in mouth

Solved

Overtired crying

Boob in mouth

Fell asleep

Woke up too soon

Crying

Few shirty looks from others
Boob in mouth
Fell back to sleep

Then, hungry at a time when there was no food given out and people were sleeping and I didn't want to bother the stewards:

Crying
Boob in mouth
Ate
Stopped crying
Slept

Turbulence
Screaming
Boob in mouth
Stopped screaming

And so on.

Don't get me wrong, I also walked up and down the aisless a lot and made more straw animals than I knew was humanly possible. But the flight was fine. And my boobs were partly, if not pretty much fully, to thank for that. That, and Dee blagging our way into the airport-roof swimming pool in Singapore for free. So refreshing.

So piss off, people. Go worry about some real problems and leave my boobs alone. In fact, it might work on other people if I just stick my boob in their mouth too. Might try it next time someone starts getting aggy. Sorry, what did you say? Oh, my boob's in your mouth, can't talk?

2 NOVEMBER

1 year 7 months

3 p.m.

First morning here was jet-lagged. Bit like a hangover, jet lag with a kid is *hard*. Little One woke up at two a.m. totally awake and ready for action. We're squeezed into a flat with another woman who we didn't want to wake up. So Dee got dressed and took Little One to the park by the beach for two hours. From two a.m. to four a.m. In torchlight. Playing in the dark. Before he went out, he said he was petrified someone would see him. Or arrest him. When I woke up, all he could talk about was joggers. Women joggers. 'Everywhere Hollie, everywhere.'

Where we live, no one gets up at four a.m. unless it's to work. Here, by the beautiful Bronte Beach, there are swarms of early risers. And the ones I've seen all seem to be female. All seem to be in Lycra, running up and down stone steps and across sandy paths and being shouted at by huge, screaming muscled men.

On the walk to the local café there are ads Blu-tacked up the sides of walls like wallpaper. A lot of fitness ones. Open-air fitness training. Lots of women on the posters. Lots of opportunities to 'get in shape', or 'get back in shape' on the ones targeting mums. And there's quite a few of those.

It makes me feel a bit unfit seeing people jogging round here all the time. But not enough to make me want to join them. Definitely not if I'm gonna get shouted at by a man who seems so angry that someone's sit-ups are 'NOT GOOD ENOUGH!' In fact, it makes me feel more relaxed that I'm totally not into that.

I'd worried about my body for a while, thought about doing that sort of rigorous training, normally after seeing someone really fit on telly or reading an article in a glossy magazine. But seeing those women, up at five a.m., running up and down, squatting, sweating for dear life as the sun rises and the instructor stands beaming like a beacon of military power, I realise it's totally not for me. I'd rather sleep or read a book. Or do exercise without being spat on. But each to their own.

My first urge when I saw some of the women was to scream: 'What the fuck are you doing? Go to sleep! Do something you love!' Then I realise, who the hell am I? Maybe running around squatting till you cry *is* what they love. Getting the fresh air, getting fit. I mean, they look in pain, but that's another thing some people love. Being in pain. Pushing their bodies to the limits.

I *try* to think that. But I just can't help feeling that part of it, for some of them at least, may possibly be to do with the pressure to get back again a body that has given birth. Even more than in the UK, where getting the opportunity to walk down a beach in a bikini is much less likely.

And that makes me glad, for the first time in my life, that I don't live in a hot country. I mean, not *really* hot. Not most of the time. I'd love it to be a bit warmer. But with a near-two-year-old kid, I am glad. Living in a cold country means that I do not often think about bikinis. Here, however, on the beaches of Sydney, I realise that for new mums there are the same body-image obsessions our media have, but combined with the bikini surf culture of the city. That must be pretty hard.

I find it hard wearing a bikini, here at least. Which is stupid. Some people are dying. I really need to get over this. People can do what they want. As long as it really is what they want.

Some Thoughts on Beauty Advertising

I know you think I'm ugly
You tell me every day
I know you say my face is rough
And not fit to parade
I know you say my skin tones
Need smoothed in creams and paint

I know you say my lips are limp
Not ripe enough to love
I know you say my laughter lines
Need needle-pumped with drugs
I know you say my wider hips
Are too damn hard to hug
And I know you said the same
About the features of my mum

I know you say our breasts need stripped
With scalpels, knives and cuts
I know you say our face and necks
need sliced and lifted up

I know you think we're ugly
Because you tell us every day
That our skins and shapes are wrong
as age sweeps us away

I know you say that I need 'fixed'
since I took upon a woman's shape
But I swear to God I will beat you down
If you tell my child the same.

1 year 8 months

Colours

Sometimes I think people
must've never seen
the colour green.

Mixed blue
with yellow on a palette
Sat back and sighed at
how beautiful it is
to have more
than three
colours
in this world, not

just
Yellow, Blue and Red

Sometimes I think people
must've never curled
a paintbrush

round a bend
seen indigo or
turquoise blends
orange, brown
or purple trends

just
Yellow, Blue and Red

I think a lot of what
Alice Walker said
contemplate how
the gardens here
the beaches
the clifftop views
the seaweed caught
between your toes
would glow
if we never mixed
things up a bit
dipped our feet
coldly in

just
Yellow, Blue and Red.

Set in Primary solidity
no mixtures please
three coloured blobs
on separate plates
of paint
splitting rainbow rays

into the most
basic set of shades.

just
Yellow Blue and Red

When people ask me
if the little girl
with me
who holds my hand
and calls me Mum
and walks along
the beach with me
is mine

I wonder if they've
ever seen sunshine
split through raindrops
or stopped to watch how
paint morphs
into new shades
every time you
stroke the brush
across a page.

One thing I've noticed here – apart from the fact that it is beautiful and warm and sunny and welcoming and a bit like having a holiday in paradise, walking across the beach clifftops – is that it's very pale. I mean, not actually pale: people are bronzed sun-dwelling god and goddess surfers where we're staying. Not pale like me. Just pale like very white. Caucasian. So Caucasian that to get his hair cane rowed for less than about £200 Dee had to sit on a train all day until he saw 'stations with brown-skinned people getting off'. With each stop out of the Sydney city centre, the hair-dressing prices went down by about fifty dollars. He got off near the end of the line. His hair looked very good.

Perhaps for this reason, it has also been one of the first places where people have questioned whether my daughter is my own or not. Openly. Frankly, like 'Is that your daughter?' whilst continually telling me how much she 'doesn't look at all like you'. It happens in England too. Since she was born, people have been saying how much she looks like Dee and not like me; but here even more so, and a bit more unashamedly related to skin colour.

I find it all a bit annoying, but interesting. I don't really know why it's something people even say, why they don't think it might be offensive – so perhaps, maybe, just don't bother!

My daughter is a pretty close middle ground between me and Dee, skin-colour-wise, hair-texture-wise, personality-wise. But of course, in mainly Caucasian-toned areas, everyone tells me she has his skin tone, because everything not 'white' is lumped together. When we're with Caucasian people, they mainly say she is the same colour as him, although on a paint palette chart it's a pretty even mix. It also varies by season and sun exposure.

On the other hand, with Dee's family, they often say the opposite. Because she's light to them, she therefore has my colouring. Same with hair texture. She has my 'soft hair'. Here, she has Dee's 'curly hair'. It's interesting how much our perspectives rely so little on fact and so much more on surroundings and comparison. With this, anyhow.

I'd love to go to a different country, with a dark-brown-skinned majority, to see if it's the same there. I think it would be. I mean, I don't need her to look like me, it really is OK. I'm just getting bored with the same statement and the reply I always give when people say 'She looks nothing like you' or 'She doesn't look like your child at all.' Seriously, this palette is not that uncommon any more. But here, maybe, it is?

After a second week here, I have a real urge to change my response.

I might just say: 'No, she's not mine. I stole her.'
And leave it at that.
Anyway, she's got my feet.

Angel

You're the most beautiful kid in the world
But the angels do not look like you
You're the most blissful vision I've seen in my days
But the angels are not in your hue
You're the reason I threw the Bible away
You're the reason I don't close my eyes when they pray
As the angels are pale-faced, blonde and blue-eyed
You are the reason I've thrown their teachings aside
Because
There is angel in your curly brown hair
There is angel in your caramel face
There is angel in your dark-soil eyes
There is angel in your quickening pace.
So
Walk away
Little kid
Walk away
From the martyrs, the angels, the saints
Walk away, little kid, walk away
From the pens and the paper and paints
Walk away, little kid, from the praise
Until Jesus is drawn in truer dark shades
Until the colonised faces are not so cheap
Until angels in museums in large gilded frames
look just like you when you sleep

4 NOVEMBER

1 year 7 months

Miles and Sarah and Billy are the greatest family to have hooked up with here. Blue Mountains and the Australian Poetry Slam in one week. And the fact they also have three different skin tones between them. Solidarity in numbers.

But I'm not writing about that. In fact, I'm not writing. It's too busy to write here. So many gigs and walks and beaches. I'm gonna take photos instead. Sometimes I just get overwhelmed with views. Writing's OK, but it sure as hell has its limitations. Sometimes I wish I was better at taking photographs.

I might never come back here in my life. I'm going out. Put the pen down Hollie, put it down.

1 year 8 months

Grandparent Love

I'm done with the love songs
of young girls and boys
of pretty-faced couples
weddings and joy

of boardwalks and beaches
and first-kiss delights
of virgin-loss sex songs
and passionate nights

I'm bored with the
monopolisation of love
by monogamous couples
and white flying doves

The one man one woman
is too overrated
Every song, every film
Every romantic statement

Couples in rain kissing
Couples in bed kissing
Couples in love kissing
Everything else missing

Watching her lips quiver
as she stared up above
cheeks stained in tears
as she grabbed for my mum

A hug that outdid any
Hollywood moulding
Just a grandma and grandchild
and ten minutes' holding

her hands to her cheeks
in eye-to-eye stares
a romantic love scene
we hardly see anywhere

as love is defined
in the narrowest ranges
and fit kissing couples
given too high a status

I want more of Vandross
dancing with his father again
and grandparent love
to reach the Top Ten

Having a child is too much. It's too emotional for me to handle. I've never been very showy with my emotions but this mum malarkey is pushing it out of me more and more.

The flight back from Australia was fine. I could manage it. Nearly a full day occupying a child in an aeroplane was nothing compared to the look on Little One's face today when she saw my mum after being away for five weeks: tears in her eyes; the most genuinely overjoyed smile I have seen in my entire life; tears in my mum's eyes at seeing the effect she had on this small bundle of lusciousness. A perfect romantic movie scene.

Since Little One was born, Mum has been making the five-hour round trip to ours every single week, Sundays and Mondays, taking Little One to toddler group, on picnics, through mud, in puddles, sitting under trees for hours picking grass. All that good stuff. Not because she has the time, she doesn't. She works near-sixty-hour weeks as a nurse jammed into the other four weekdays, plus most Saturdays on top of that now that the government seems to think medical staff don't need weekends or days off any more. So in those smidgens of free time, she gets in a car, drives two hours to us, plays in parks, cleans our cooker and gets woken up at six a.m. instead of us the next morning. I think it is because she is an angel. I think that's it. And, she says, because she doesn't want me to be as tired as she was.

Today was so beautiful. Mum has been constantly worrying she's interfering too much, coming up to visit too much, asking me continually if it's OK for her to come, if I find it annoying. I don't know where she gets this from. I don't know how many times I can tell her that her visits are one of the highlights of my life at the minute, one of the most helpful things anyone has done for me and Dee both; that I love seeing her. I'm the one who should be worrying about all her journeys, time, petrol money. But she's still questioning me.

So seeing her reaction as Little One looked into her eyes after a five-week separation and physically broke down was a delight. The grandmas have worked so hard to forge these relationships. My mum, Dee's mum too. For Dee's mum, it has been nearly a year of us dropping off Little One one day a week at her house and Little One screaming and crying all day long during the visit and her still saying 'Please bring her round next week again, it's fine.' They are magical grandmas. Magical, working, busy, selfless, beautiful grandmas. If I ever become one, I hope I'm on that level.

1 year 8 months

It's freezing outside, the trees are bare and the local lake is frosting. I've been spending quite a lot of time with Little One throwing sticks on the lake to crack the ice and make the ducks some liquid paths to pass through. Little One is loving the game.

But today was too cold. We went to a mate's instead. It's so lovely having friends I can now phone and say 'We're just passing, are you in for a cuppa?' To be honest, half the time I'm not passing. I just walk somewhere close by or get in the car so I have the excuse. I'm not at the 'We've got nothing to do and I really, really want some company, can I please come and hang at your house with you and your kids and drink tea?' stage yet. One day, maybe.

Sitting sipping tea watching cartoons is so nice sometimes. On top of that, I saw the Coca-Cola Christmas advert, which means Christmas is officially on its way. I know it's a marketing jingle, but it has worked on me. It is firmly set in my Christmas nostalgia brain, alongside decorating the tree, driving to Gran's house, eating Mum's and then Aunt Jan's potatoes and stuffing, and opening my presents slowly enough so I would have a few left after my brother was done opening his. That was hard, 'cos he opens presents slowly, savours each one. He gets a present, it's a book, he makes a drink and reads the whole fucking thing. Music album, he's up in his room to hear every godamn track. It was a killer. He still does the same – I do too. I mean, I wait for him, hiding presents behind my back for hours.

Anyway, Coca-Cola is here and that means it is Christmas now. I vividly remember when I was little asking my dad why there wasn't a TV channel where I could watch adverts all day. I loved adverts, like I loved music videos. Little snippets of TV genius. And Christmas did not feel like Christmas until I saw the Coca-Cola advert with the train and the 'Holidays are coming' song. Not for me, not for half the country. I didn't get what adverts were really, so didn't understand why an advert channel wouldn't work or why a child forcibly associating the joy of Christmas and holidays and happiness with a fizzy drink full of nothing but shite, rotting the nation's teeth, is possibly not a great thing.

For the last few years I've not had a TV, so I've not seen any adverts. I forgot what, apart from the Coke lorry, Christmas ads were like. Sitting at a mate's house, watching Little One stare at the screen as the toy ads flash before her, is like watching a weird experiment. Adverts are so loud, so exciting, so flashy. I don't know what it was like in my toddlerhood 'cos I can't remember, but it's amazing the difference between the boys' and girls' Christmas ads. Guns for boys, beauty for girls. Even Lego has split into grenades and glitter – a few 'City' sets for both, but mainly now separate. I understand why Lego, and most other companies have started to do this. It sells twice the products – stops siblings sharing toys and discourages hand-me-downs between the sexes, so more money for the brand. Economically, it is genius. Socially and culturally, it is pretty sad. And having now spent a lot of time with actual small children, I find it astonishing the way, even now, people increasingly treat, dress, hold and talk to boys and girls differently. Even as babies.

One of the teenage boys in our poetry workshops killed himself last month. My mum always used to tell me about her patients at Christmas and New Year. How suicide is rife in holidays like that. Because the expectations are so high, unhappiness is harder to bear, I guess. And it's meant to be perfect. Surrounded by family and gifts and love and fulfilment and beautiful lit up Coca-Cola lorries delivering help and happiness to all who come into its shining path. He was so shy. So quiet. It's so fucking sad.

I watch the Christmas adverts fill my daughter's 'I want that', 'that will make me happy in life', greed-inducing brain portion and sip tea. I love sitting on the couch and chatting. But the adverts make me a little sick after a while.

Poetry

At the workshops he was too shy to join in
there's always one like him –
Others chorusing their thoughts
over creative exercise plans;
their A-Z of favourite bands
or words
or colours
scribbling lines on paper
we'd soon make into poems
sitting together – one large circle now – in the hall
trying to work out how to make anger fall in ink
what happiness would taste like if you drank it
how freedom might sound if you could hear it

It always upsets me how much teenagers
have upon their shoulders
– family, exams, homeless, sex, violence, stress –
It always carves onto the page or to their skin

He peeked around the corner
never coming in
We tried to coax him with
soft voices
and patience

and tea
left the pen and pad easily placed in his reach
– just in case –
he felt like setting fingers free
He smiled at me once through teenage curtained hair
hung down

The worker stayed with him
encouraging
never giving up on him
till the very end
of class

I'm always amazed how young people
have such a lot to say
but are seldom ever, ever asked to speak

They sent us an email the next week
to thank us for the day
said that the young boy
in the kitchen
had tried to kill himself again
and this time
unfortunately
had made it;

faded into the silence
he so wished
to hide in.

It always empties guts
into my mouth

when the world is not enough
when the flowers aren't enough
when the birds can't sing loud enough
when the sun cannot rise high enough
when the grass cannot grow green enough
when the rainbow does not glow enough
when words cannot deep-clean enough
to keep a young kid keen enough
when his tongue will not allow him
to shout loud enough
or his fingers
spill the ink
enough
to let him get it out of him
and live

My mum always sipped her tea a little quieter at home
when patients commited suicide
would roll her eyes
instead of cry
and whisper to the steam
If only they had waited
I'm sure they would've seen
if only they had waited
if only
she would say.

They said he had enjoyed the day.
The tea.
The writing.
The poetry.

Christmas Adverts

Pink
It's all bollocks
Blue
It's all bollocks

Babygros for boys with robots on
Babygros for girls – no robots on
Babygros for boys with trains on
Babygros for girls – no trains on
It's all bollocks

Tops for little girls with love hearts on
Tops for little boys – no love hearts on
Tops for little girls with sparkles on
Tops for little boys – no sparkles on
It's all bollocks

Little girls given ballet shoes
Little boys given football boots
Little girls told they can point with toes
Little boys told they can kick with toes
It's all bollocks

Little girls told they are princesses – need saving
Little boys told they are knights – need to save
        them
Princesses – bollocks
Knights – bollocks
Pressure to fight – bollocks

Little boys given guns – told to shoot
Little girls given jewellery – told to look cute
Shoot – bollocks
Cute – bollocks

Little girls with tears in their eyes – given hugs
Little boys with tears – told to man up
stand up
stiffen up
harden up
suck it up
toughen up
it's all bollocks

boys sold Lego rockets
girls sold Lego lockets
boys told not to cry – bollocks
girls told not to fight – bollocks

teenage girls having sex – slag
teenage boy having sex – lad
teenage girls having no sex – prude
teenage boy having no sex – loser
teenage girls acting tough – soften
teenage boys acting soft – rotten

Boys told to man up
Girls told to make up
boys told to stand up
girls told to shut up
boys told to be tough
girls told to be pretty

men told to make money
women told to stay pretty
men told to be strong
women told to stay young
men having breakdowns
women having Botox
men having crises
women having vaj jobs
men told to be rich
women told to be thin
women told they need saved
men told to save them
women told to be ladies
do not spit or shout or smell
men told to be a man
do not cry or ask for help
men having breakdowns
women having Botox
young boys committing suicide
young girls ripping their pubes off
young boys trying to live up to
Superhero action figures
young girls trying to live up to
Beauty Barbie stick-thin figures

Boys told to be more
Girls told to be less

Babygros with knights on
or Babygros with princesses.

1 year 9 months

Your Face

Your face makes people calmer
and your smile makes them realise
that most worries do not matter
in this life
much.

Your face makes people beam
and your laughter seems to
highlight how most of our
morals are quite
messed up.

My grandma moment came today. Being in Scotland in winter reminds me of being heavily pregnant now; those cold winds that cooled my heavy belly, the stolen grabs of snow or hail shoved into my craving mouth; and Gran. Gran's wedding ring in particular. Gran's wedding ring continually attempted to be slipped onto my finger on public outings.

The first visit to see Gran after having Little One was amazing. She was so worried when I was pregnant, and it often made me feel a little crap about myself. She'd mention marriage a lot and how I should do that so that Little One would not be born a bastard. That word sounded harsh at the time. She also worried about the fact Little One would be 'mixed race'. All these things look pretty prejudiced on paper.

In reality they were just the reaction of a person brought up three generations ago in a culture that taught women that their pregnant bodies – in or out of wedlock – were a shameful, even disgusting, sight; that sex was an obligatory sin for a married woman to undergo; that sex and babies out of wedlock were the Devil's work and that mixed-race children would be confused and bullied. Nothing she said to me was out of anything but love and worry; she was worried Little One would be picked on for her skin tone and for her unmarried parents. She was petrified that this small human, who she had not even met yet, would be bullied in later years. She was being loving, protective. Of me and of the unborn baby. And where *she* comes from, the place and the time, that was a likely thing that would've happened. I think that is true love, really. I shouldn't take offence at any of it. I'm just glad that I was born two generations after that.

Me and my gran have talked a lot about these things, about how social conventions and ideas and morals have changed a lot since she was a new mum – not enough, but quite a lot. The thing I love most about her is that as soon as she saw Little One, she seemed to forget all this baggage of social ideas – to shun it, even. Shun years of ideas firmly rooted in her upbringing. She just saw a smiling, happy baby. Not a bastard; not an unchristened sinner; not the fact her skin was a different hue to my own. Just a gorgeous, smiling child. Everyone around me just saw a smiling happy baby. I wish everyone could see that. It makes me want to weep that even babies are judged in so many ways. For their skin; 'status'; their place of birth even.

Today was one of the most emotional parts of this journey with my gran. We sat down to have a tea and a Tunnock's as Little One slumped napping in the back bedroom. Gran handed me a cheque for two hundred pounds and said: 'You're a great mum with a beautiful child and partner. I know you don't want to get married and I've accepted that, so this is the money I gave to each of your cousins on their wedding day.'

I think this is a big deal. A big enough deal that it made me sob for a good hour once I was out of Gran's sight. For an eighty-year-old woman who believes deeply in marriage to say and do this – well, I think it's kind of proof that my gran is fucking amazing.

It's also got me thinking about whether I could get a honeymoon at some point, or at least the equivalent of a cheap wedding dress, off my parents. I am saving people a lot of money here. A new toaster, just?

26 DECEMBER

1 year 9 months

I don't want to do that to myself again
I thought that I would die
It's like opting for a car crash
a second time
just because the aftercare was grand

I love my child.
I love my lonely, only child
I love the fact I trampolined today without weeing in my pants

The ultimate joke this Christmas: *Aren't you going to get her a little brother or sister as a present? Maybe for her birthday? Next Christmas?*

The pressure to have another child has been ramped up since Little One turned one, with the added excitement of warnings about how she will be lonely, spoilt, bored, frustrated etc. without siblings. I get it. I totally love my brother. He's a beautiful, beautiful person and a great friend and support. But so are my friends. And my cousins. So I will make sure she has friends and cousins close by.

The only person on my side – apart from Dee, Mum and Dad, who don't give a toss, which is great – is Dee's grandma Ionie. She whispered to me over dinner, 'I had seven, can you imagine? We couldn't really say no in those days. Stick with one, love, 'cos you can.' I really love her sometimes.

The pressure to have a kid in the first place was bad enough. My friends complain a lot about this pressure that's put on them to have children. I need to tell them that having a child won't appease it, so think carefully! I thought that after having one kid that would stop, but now people just want another, and I realise there will always be more and more that people want from you and you will never really meet expectations. My flat will always be too small, my finger unringed, job not stable enough, salary not high enough, hair not sleek enough, legs not smooth enough – whatever it is. So I will just chill and leave people to worry about my life and smile when asked when the next one's coming.

I have tried lots of different replies this past year:

Because I don't want another one (this is selfish, because it is not about what *I* want any more).

Because I don't want to be pregnant or give birth again (this is selfish, because the first birth was fine and it's not about me).

Because I feel I'm only just getting back a life of my own now and I fucking love it (this is selfish, because it's all me, me, me).

Because I can't (this totally shuts people up. There is no response to it. It made me feel bad, though – because for some people it's true, and for me it's not. That was a last resort on a bad day. But it did make me think how rude and intrusive it is to ask people that question – you never ever know why people make the choices they do).

Apart from the jokes and light-hearted pressure, Christmas was so lovely. Having a child at Christmas makes me remember what it's like to feel that magic again. And how much I love to lie – otherwise known as telling stories or using your imagination. I love lying about Santa and telling the St Nicholas story. I really love the lies. Not so keen on the virgin-obsessive side of this celebration – have started referring to them as Virgin Mary and Virgin Joseph to get a bit of balance there! But the story about the old man giving a present to every child in the world – *one* present to *every* child, not just to a new king – that story, I like.

I realise that part of my job as a parent is making memories. Sneaking in to fill the stocking, choosing the juiciest satsuma for the toe-point reach of it, the chocolate pennies, the reindeer food and mince pies. I got a bit obsessed with it all this year. I want to create excellent memories for Little One: cook food she will smell in twenty years' time and be reminded of our evenings together; get the scratchy woollen fabric of the stocking just right so that just getting her nail snagged in a thread will remind her of Christmas Day for evermore. That's one of my favourite memories of Christmas as a kid.

Other people don't seem as concerned to do this. Sitting watching TV seems to be good enough. But I want carol-singing memories and the-smell-of-mulled-cider-wafting-through-the-air memories and – ach, never mind. I'm a bit panicky that this is not possible and far too influenced by films like *Home Alone*. I'm also starting to realise the immense amount of work and time and love and frustration that must've gone into making these life memories of mine, Christmas ones, birthday ones, weekend and holiday and everyday ones. It's a tough job and I want to get it right.

Behind the Scenes

I don't remember the time you spent
wrapping crinkled paper up with ribbons
helter skelter spirals
from that shiny thin party string
curled around the scissors' edge
Sellotape and name tags

piled upon your bed
till three a.m.

I don't remember that

I remember the tree stacked
and unwrapping sparkly gifts
on Christmas Day

I don't remember the time you sat
and stared into space
placing piles of cards and envelopes up
in strange midnight towers
hand stuck for hours
in a pen hold
teeth gritted
scribbling the neighbours' names
and holiday messages from all of us
the taste of the envelope
stuck to your tongue

I don't remember that

I remember the deliveries done
running to post them through letterboxes in the cold
and glowing excitedly opening all the Christmas cards we got

I don't remember the kitchen being hot
or the panic that the taste would not be good enough
or the hours you spent cutting up the veg, alone,
flicking frantically through recipes
as we sat lazy lounge throne chiefs

watching shit TV
as you poured more cups of tea
and prepared us snacks

I don't remember that

I remember being called when everything was ready
The smell of gravy poured on creamy mash
and disguising turnip hash with delicious apple sauce
more custard drowning out a crumble
I don't remember being made.

My childhood life – a stage
with you behind the scenes

Now I'm down there in the rigging
it's not as easy as it seemed.

1 year 10 months

I've been asked to write a poem by a breastfeeding group. They asked me to take all the phrases that mums have given them about what it's like to be a parent and patch it into a poem. I've not done anything like this, but I give it a go. It's quite long, too long, but I don't have time to edit it. I'll just send it and hope for the best.

What's My Name Again?

I lost my name
at toddler group

From Hollie, or Hols or Hobbit or Hollie McNish
I'm now known as 'so-and-so's mum'
And I cannot complain
'Cos I'm just the same
I put this same label on everyone

I met Izzy's dad for a drink at the park
we bumped into Molly's gran
and Tiana's and Mark's
and it's only when the stars are out and everything's dark

and it's night and she's finally fallen asleep
that my name label creeps out from under the table
and I am able to remember the person I am
with a hot cup of tea and a book in my hand
and a two-hour slot to remember my own plans
before I turn off my light.

Cinderella's clock strikes at midnight each time
My clock strikes loudly at nine.

Now it's your time, it chimes,
and my name becomes Hollie once more.
Until she cries out for me
or needs her next wee
or shouts in her dreams
or pleads for a fiftieth cuddle from me
or I sneak into her room just to look at her sleep
and the label shifts quickly to mum again.

To mum again.
From Hollie to Mum
From Hollie to Mum
Like a grandfather clock
or a metronome run
a life-raising swing
between structure and fun

But one word cannot sum up
The things we've all done
The way that we love
The stories we tell

As she asks me for stories in queues and on trains
in cars and by lakes as we sit
sipping on days that
we mould for our kids
who don't give a shit
about the style of our clothes
our grand lack of sleep
or our hairs turning grey
as we worrier warriors structure our days
into play –
building dens from pegged shirts
dirty and snot-striped
as sleeves wipe their noses
no bouquets of roses are thrown on our stages

underpaid, overworked

Us feeders
us nappy-change divas
us breeders
us milk-makers
milk-strainers
cracked-nipple swell painful
bottle-fed
guilt-ridden
time-giving
minds riddled all day and night with their care
one o'clock in the morning
just to check they are fine
if the covers are on right
if the nappy is too tight
if the bedroom is too light

so that even in the middle of a mother's own night
she's not quite an individual in her own right

But she's strong
craving her own space
and told that that's wrong
A sleepless survivor that longs just to lie down
to have a wee on her own
or a bath by herself
who sometimes feels like
she's given herself
for this role

In a land where we are now known as so-and-so's dad
or thingamy's mum
A label that's filled with more love
than I ever knew.

Someone said mums are the rocks that never crumble.
I don't think that's true.
'Cos I do.
I cry hidden in loos
I scream alone in my car
and when I'm woken once more
and desperate to sleep
I weep watching the stars
and every mum that I know says those moments are never so far.

We are parents but we are people
We are snot-rags and we are dreamers
We are queens and we are cleaners
We are kissed and we are screamed at

We are sleep-deprived gardeners, cut hands hidden in gloves.
We are rocks crumbling sometimes in love that's so heavy.

We are story-telling experts.
And our stories are many.

10

SPRING
TWO YEARS OLD
'THE TERRIBLE TWOS'

10 MARCH

Nearly 2 years old

6 p.m.

It amazes me how quickly people can judge you on a single glimpse of your life. As if from that small moment of your existence they can guess everything about you, what you are like and, more importantly, what sort of parent you are.

Today, I went to the market. I love taking Little One there. We buy cheap veg and she scoffs the free bread, biscuits, olives, carrots and everything else her cute face gets handed from all the sellers we've seen most weeks since she was born.

We walk around town and listen to the buskers. I love how, while everyone else just stands gormlessly in front of musicians, kids let their bodies lead, dancing in the street unashamedly to any beat they might hear. No alcohol required. I love it when Little One gets excited by buskers. When she really focuses on someone playing music like she's switched off and fallen into a trance. Partly because I feel she's soaking up brilliant life notes and that if anything has a point on this huge piece of rock, it's music. Live music especially. Partly also because it means I can sit on my arse while she dances for half an hour to a teenager playing the trumpet in the middle of town.

So we eat and laugh and listen to music and dance and toddle about town holding hands. Romantic. A free day out in the sun. Until she flips. Until I tell her we have to quickly drop the bags off in the car before we go to the park. And she flips.

I muster my calm, collected, 'I watched *Supernanny* on repeat the whole way through my pregnancy and am a good parent' attitude. I get down to her level and say in that low-toned, calm, annoying fucking voice that grates on me and Dee almost as much as it does her: 'We will just go to the car, drop off the bags and then walk to the park.'

At which points she pushes me, shouting full pelt in the middle of the busy street and lies on the floor screaming and wailing at me. She will not move. She has morphed her body into a rag doll with no bones or muscle.

I feel my face going a bit red. I stay calm. Look to the sky. I sit next to her, my arm on her back, as she wails and screams and my face gets slightly hotter and redder as every single person that walks past seems to stare deep into my wretched soul. If I pick her up, it'll be worse and Supernanny will possibly film me and make me sit and watch my own failure over and over again on repeat later on. So I just sit and wait it out.

As I sit awkwardly smiling to passers-by, a man drunk as a skunk points at us from across the street and starts to sing 'You're not old enough to have a child.' Over and over again. Perfect. Lush. Thanks. People walk past, smirk, look sorry for me or disapprovingly at me. I overthink their glances. They are just glancing because I am the lead part in a drunk man's song and my child is screaming in a place where people tend not to do that so early into the day.

Forget that rational thinking. Right now, I am making up their thoughts, constructing their idea of me in my head. I stupidly look down at myself, judging every aspect of my appearance: my earrings; the tracksuit I am wearing; my trainers; the plastic bags my shopping is bulging out of. A woman walks past. She's very smart. No plastic bags, just a Waitrose tote. I should dress more like her, perhaps. Pencil skirt, blouse. Do my hair better. I re-tie my ponytail. I'd look stupid in her outfit, though. And there is nothing wrong with a tracksuit. Comfort and pockets.

So I'll just sit on the pavement of a busy street taking in every passing stare as my child screams at me and a man tattoos his drunken shouts into the far-reaching corners of my heart.

Then she stops.

He shouts across the street some more:

'You're not old enough to have a kid.'

She starts again. Everyone stares at me again. He continues standing, pointing and shouting louder now:

'LOOK AT YOU! YOU ARE NOT FUCKING OLD ENOUGH TO HAVE A KID! YOU SHOULD NOT HAVE A KID!'

Ground, please swallow me up. I've clicked my heels ten times but nothing. Where the fuck is Kansas when you need it?

I'm not sure I have ever felt so low in my entire life. I know it's OK. No one is hurt. Still, I jerk back tears. If I cry, I'll look like an idiot. If I cry, he'll think I've proved his point. If I cry, Little One will cry more. If I cry, someone will ask if I'm all right in sympathetic tones that imply I am the worst mum on this earth and desperately need a hand to just look after one small child. So I sit on the street and wait it out. Keep calm and repeat over and over in my head:

The man is blind drunk
The people will pass by
They do not know me
They only know this moment
It doesn't matter
You're a good mum, Hollie
It doesn't matter what people think
Shake it off
It doesn't matter
They don't even actually care
It's all in your head.

The tantrum lasted all of eight minutes and the rest of the day was beautiful:

Grass to roll in.

Swings.

Kissing in the sunshine.

Climbing trees.

Feeding ducks.

Stories.

That night I kissed her forehead as she fell asleep, smiling at me as she did. She is lovely. I left the room and spent the next hour sobbing into a sofa cushion. Wine downed. Breathe out.

Judgement is draining, no matter how mistaken you know people are about you. No matter how much it's just your own ideas. I still want a T-shirt that says 'You don't know me. Do not judge me on this tiny moment.'

2 years old

9 p.m.

The Terrible Twos: 1

Now you can walk and now you can run
Now that new words drip each day from your tongue
Now that your mind wants to think for itself
Now your opinions are developing strength
Now that your thoughts become independent
Your brain conceiving its first self-reflections
Now that your dreams are beginning to grow
Now that your own self is starting to show
Now that your confidence is swelling each day
And all baby-like features are floating away
Now your emotions are making new moves
We complain and claim it's the 'terrible twos'
Our first shitty label for small humankind
The minute they start to know their own minds

Since Little One has turned two, everything she does other than smiling or hugging, I'm told, is because of 'the Terrible Twos'. When she screams or cries or gets frustrated or angry: 'Oh no, it's the Terrible Twos.' I'm getting sick of it. *I* scream. *I* cry. *I* get frustrated then angry then upset then happy and sometimes all at once – and I'm twenty-eight, for God's sake. I've got way more experience than she has. I've had way more time to work myself out. I'm starting to feel sorry for toddlers. So far, I'm loving the Terrible Twos a lot more than I remember loving the newborn 'phase'. I hate the phrase 'Terrible Twos' – it's so dismissive. Just because they are no longer keeping as quiet and as still. And yeah, it can be terrible. But to scar a whole year from the beginning is excessive. I know a hell of a lot of grumpy, moody, indecisive, tantrum-prone adults.

The Terrible Twos: 2

Toddlers – and teenagers
– let's treat them like shit
Warn every parent about this age of barred bliss
Label any new emotion 'moods'
and proclaim as they push their food away
that that's just how this awful age range *all* behave.

Toddlers and teenagers, so similar in some respects
Toddlers and teenagers, so much more deserving of respect
They've learnt to make their own mixed thoughts
and now they want to rule their heads
through hormone shifts and new found senses
they learnt to walk alone
and now they want to use their legs

To run a bit away, a little bit, from us.

And we say
'Troublemakers',
'Tantrums',
'Mood swings',
'Selfish',
'Sulky',
'Hard',
'Unruly'.
Making truly shitty pictures
of terrible twos and rude teenagers
we place our labels on their ages
red marks already rule their pages
as they both try so very hard
to work out who on earth they are

And we cry
'Tantrums!'
'Traumas!'
'Trouble!'
because they create a little rubble
as they step away a little
push the boundaries of the bubbles
that we made

They want to play
to walk the other way a bit
a bit too far away for us
and see how far the edge can stretch
until it stops for them one day
as my two-year-old takes off her clothes
in the middle of the shop again
and asks me 'Why?'

when I say no
and then stops everyone around us
as she screams
for ice-cream.
Please.
'No,' I say, again
so she repeats a little louder
'Ice-cream *please.*'

So
now she's
crying on the floor
pleading, grabbing both my knees
and we try to stay calm as we can
while everyone around us looks
but it's us who made them all this food
it's us who made the ice-cream
it's us who added sugared treats
to every kids' food factory
and they really wanted more of it
learning how to deal with 'Noes'
beating hands on broken floors
battling frustration's claws
for the first time in their life
working out reactions
and grasping anger's knife

So they hide in dens and under hoods
creating worlds in woods and books
as they look to other things to guide them
outside the scan of adults eyes
and we cry

'Troublemakers!'
'Tantrums!'
'Stress!'

proclaim they're trying it all to test us
proclaim they need a good firm lesson
to get them back in tow

as they try so very hard to safely let us go
and make their own rough-weeded path
stepping slowly day by day
a little further from our grasp.

2 years 1 month

11 p.m.

Right now, Little One is obsessed with going outside, making bows and arrows and reading. I love it. Mainly down to our park visits, as well as inspired by the films *Beauty and the Beast* and *Brave*. I know people who don't like Disney, but I love a lot of the stories, the music, the animation. *Brave* is the newest film, featuring a Disney princess named Merida. The fact that the film is set in Scotland meant that my mum and dad had bought it as a present for Little One before I'd even heard of it. But I like it. A princess who is far removed from the shy, simpering Snow White. Although she's pretty brave too. All those thorns and rabbit's eyes. So Merida is the new figure, with flowing, but messy, hair, who doesn't want tight dresses she can't move in, who rides horses, explores the highlands, fires arrows, and most importantly, refuses to be married off as a teenager. And is Scottish. Did I say she's Scottish?

Little One loves the film. She forces me to be the horse. My gran thinks it is a bad influence on her and has been suggesting other films ever since she found me galloping across the living room, Little One on my back shouting, 'I will not marry that prince, I want to ride to the mountains.'

But today, Disney released the new-look Merida and I was a bit sad. I can handle the simpering storylines and doe eyes that trail through a lot of Disney characters, but this sexiness in kids' films is odd.

Tinkerbell. The Little Mermaid. They are all part of great storylines. Tinkerbell is an engineering tinker fairy. But they focus so much on her bum and fluttering eyes and the short-cut dress. Ariel swims a fully grown man through the waves and saves his life in a stormy sea, then must sexily flick back her hair and pose on the rocks. It's weird. It's weird to make kids' characters so sexual. *Brave* was a bit fresh. There, Merida was just drawn as a kid. A normal, adventurous kid. Now for some reason Disney has 'redone' her for all the products and posters and pictures related to the film. Not just a new dress for that princess inauguration stuff. A new Merida. A sexier Merida. I'm sick of it being seen as a necessary thing. She's sexy now, like every other picture of every other female we ever see. Just sexy. We're just sexy, that's our only role in this place. Even in kids' films. It's weird. And they've nicked her bow and arrow.

Merida

I know this is not the most important thing
and no one's gonna die from it
But this little change to me sums up
the messages that Disney gives

Where curls must all be fixed or glossy
despite the years the filmmakers took
to get the wildness of that hair
the girl who dares to climb up mountains
wailing winds to bravely follows will-o'-wisps
and couldn't give two ticks
how her hair looked
while she's doing it

But now they combed out all those bits
and she looks more like a shampoo ad
hair tossed back and shoulders slack
looking sweetly back at us.

and it is not the most important thing to fuss
        about
and no one's gonna die
and if you do not like it then yes, of course
you do not have to buy it
but I think it's also right to stand up
to million-dollar companies
who feel some weird need
to make cartoon kids
in children's films
look sexy.

And I know it's just a drawing
and you say it doesn't matter how a drawing looks
but my two-year-old's been making bows and arrows in the
        woods
and says
'this Merida is standing still
'cos she can't move in her tighter dress',
and her hair can't be a mess
and her bow is a now shiny belt
clipping in a stick-thin waist
and her face is more made up
with sexy eyelined eyes and gaze and smile
and you have made it all about her style
sexified another child
and like every other Disney princess toy,

made her wider-eyed
and coy

As the camera zooms to Tinkerbell's bum some more
and we ignore her engineering scores
your Merida is now a bore
and doesn't aim arrows any more
and cannot have a wider jaw
and needs to have a body morph
and look demurely at the camera.
I find it an embarrassment
and I know that no one's gonna die
but still we need to challenge it
because it's all a little messy
where even fairies must look sexy
and every girl must be a beauty
bat her eyes and shoulders cutely
and while the story was a hit
your marketing is stupid.

2 years 2 months

8 p.m.

I have just succeeded in taking a ten-hour train journey with a two-year-old. I want a sticker. I really want a Well Done sticker.

There are moments in life when you just want to look people in the face and say: *Why? Why are you doing this to me?* Today had moments like that. Golden moments too. Either way, I want a fucking sticker.

I have never been so organised in all my life as I was today. I booked every train around every possible daily routine Little One has.

Train to London: before first nap. Eurostar to France: during nap exactly, to the minute, with the nap hopefully lasting longer than normal, until the connecting train five hours later. For this to work, I kept her up until eleven p.m. last night. She woke up in the morning, overtired, and we got on the train to London. Snacks out. She was knackered, but no way was she sleeping on this part of the journey, otherwise the rest of the day is fucked. So I chatted and played and we ate and got to London King's Cross. Walking to Euston could've been disastrous, with the lulling of the pushchair, so I carried her. A grape in mouth every two minutes. Carried her and the pushchair and the bag. Chatted, kept her awake. So far, so good. I've always been pretty good at inane chatting.

We get through customs (she needed to be awake for this because of the checks), and the minute I'm into the departure lounge I have twenty minutes to get her to sleep. So I change her. Then I strap her in the pushchair. She cries, I kiss her, she cries and I pace around the lounge in walk–jog frantic circles, wobbling the pram from side to side in the way that for some reason helps her nod off. Keep checking her face. Not sleeping. Check again. Not sleeping. Crying. Fifteen minutes of pacing and she's out. She's sleeping. I'm a genius. The plan has worked.

I check the tickets and get to the right door of the train. Get in. Coach F.

There's a pram space in the entrance bit before the carriage. I park the pram and sit on the fold-out seat. I can't get to my actual seat, the bigger, comfier one – with a tray that I could possibly put a cup of tea on – to sit in for this four-hour journey, but I do not care. I will sit in this area surrounded by luggage and the smell of the toilets because she is asleep and I am a train journey genius and comfy seats are an overrated luxury.

Ten minutes before the train is due to leave, the train manager comes through. She looks at me and says, flippant, like it's nothing: 'You'll have to fold up the pram and put it up in the luggage compartment, madam.'

No fucking way.

No. Fucking. Way.

'But this is the pram area,' I say.

'Yes, but there's another pram in the next one so we need to put one down.'

I start to sweat. Palms, back of the knees. Nape of neck. A five-hour journey with a kid on my lap is one thing. But a five-hour journey with a kid that has been woken up from a long-overdue nap is another. I know this. She will cry. She will cry for a long, long time. The other passengers will hate me and ignore me and the train manager will not help with this. She will not say 'Oh sorry it was my fault you woke her, let me walk her up and down the corridor and make rockets out of cups for you.' She won't.

So I say 'OK' and the manager leaves but I don't fold the pram up. I take it off the train and race into the next carriage with it. Then, when I see the manager coming back our way, I pick it up again and go back to the first carriage I was in, so that she passes inside, I pass outside, at the same time. I get back into the original space and pray to the god of sleeping toddlers that the demon manager from hell isn't going to make me do what she's told me to do. The train pulls off. The manager is walking back towards us. I lay my head on the top of the pram and pretend to be fast asleep. Even sweatier now from panic, fear and exertion, I close my eyes tight shut and keep absolutely still. She passes by and away. I sit on the uncomfortable flip-seat for four hours, dreaming a little of the seat I booked and paid for. I can see it, even. But I can't move the pushchair. And she is sleeping. A numb bum is nothing compared to that.

Little One wakes up, well rested and smiling, just as I get off that train. We board the final train fifteen minutes later, step in and look around the carriage. Two people are sitting, thirty or so empty seats, and a luggage rack clear as a kids' play cage. It is like walking onto a luxury yacht. An empty carriage for the last two hours with an energetic kid. She sits in the luggage rack and plays the whole journey. I sit in a comfy seat and order a tea and look around in awe at the beauty of this empty, *empty* public space.

2 years 2 months

8 p.m.

On the way back from France, Little One falls asleep before we go through the Eurostar scanner bit. Fuck. I get to the front of the queue and say in my best French: 'I know I have to wake her to walk her through. I'll be one minute.'

I remember when we went to Australia, there was a woman going through customs with three kids. A baby and toddler sleeping in a pushchair and an older one, maybe five, walking next to her. When she got to the scanning bit, the airport staff told her she needed to take the kids out of the pushchair to go through – and to fold down the pushchair to be X-rayed. I can still picture that moment, the devastation on her face. Still, like a don, she managed to haul the sleeping toddler onto her chest, still asleep, and instructed the older child to lift up the baby. Pushchair folded and put on the conveyer belt. Not good enough. She had to wake up the toddler, so the kid could walk through the scanner, screaming grumpy. Baby also frisked. By the time she was through – no beeping or bag to search – she had three children, two screaming, and a pushchair she struggled to unfold with two kids held to her waist who were refusing to get in it. Security, I get it. Was still a tragic scene to watch.

'*Une seconde, s'il vous plaît,*' I repeat. The customs officer, or whatever the job title is, looks at me like I'm unstable, quickly interrupts me before I go to reach for Little One and says: '*Non!* Don't wake a sleeping child!' He then proceeds to body-check her in the pram and lead us through the business-class speedy boarding, skipping the queues and showing us exactly where to sit so that I can 'leave her in the pram to sleep'. Might just be a person-to-person thing, but right now, the French are winning the parent-friendly customs battle, that one man championing the whole Republic. Either that, or ingrained racism of British customs checks – that mother of three was brown-skinned and wearing a headscarf.

Little One slept nearly the entire way back to London. I sat on the flip-out seat and read a book. Numb Bum Bliss.

2 years 2 months

3 p.m.

Trains

Today someone at the Tuesday toddler group said it was strange to see Little One playing with trains so much. I explained that she comes on the train with me to work gigs all the time and loves it. She goes on the train to Scotland to see the family. We've just been to France on the train. The woman said again that it was normally little boys who play with trains and repeated, with light, friendly laughter, how strange that she liked trains. I'm hearing this sort of thing more and more now. A little boy last week was encouraged by his dad not to play with the pram and doll that are in the wendy house area. The same dad who had just pushed him to toddler group in a pram. Probably from a house, I imagine.

I've been asked five hundred times when Little One will start ballet by family because 'she points her toes so well'. Every time she plays princesses people tell me she's such a little girl. Every time she jumps in puddles and climbs trees, she's a tomboy. No, she's not. She's just a girl who sometimes likes climbing trees and sometimes likes dressing up. Just like a little boy pushing a pram is not pretending or trying to be a girl. He is just a little boy pushing a pram. She's only two and she's already being pushed and boxed and fitted into our ideas of what girls and boys should be and do.

I am slowly losing my belief that much of our behaviour is natural. Before I had a baby, I thought it was. But everything is so forced now, I'm losing that belief. It's getting harder to find books about girls and boys playing together. Everything is split. Me and Dee went to Halfords today and every single kid's bike was branded and labelled 'girls' or 'boys'. I was really excited about buying Little One a bike and I'd been imagining an excited trip with her running round the bike shop with me and Dee testing out the heights and pedalling wobbles. But I don't even want to take her into shops with me any more. I just go to the bike shop by myself, to avoid the hassle.

The bikes themselves were decorated so differently. The girls' bikes had seats for the teddy on the back and a basket on the front. Often glittery. Often with sparkly pom pom things stuck out the handle bars. There were no baskets for the little boys' bikes or teddy seats or exciting sparkling decorations – as if little boys would never want to take their toys out or pick blackberries or collect conkers on a bike ride. There was a little boy asking for a basket in the shop. All the baskets were pink and the shop keeper was telling him how they didn't have boys baskets. Gutted. The boys' bikes were all quite dull colours, but decorated with 'speed' – lightning flashes and all that stuff. The girls' bikes had no lightning, no police, no speed – princesses mainly, and seemed to say 'potter around on me, collect things, take teddy for a ride, be a princess on me'. The boys bikes screamed 'speed, adventure, cycle me, race me – but don't bring your beloved teddy, 'cos that's soppy and far too loving and sweet'. Even the height charts were separated. The boys' one had dinosaurs and robots on it, the girls' one ballerinas and princesses. I told a little boy today that the dinosaur he was playing with was a grandma. He laughed and said, 'No it's not!' I picked it up and started talking to him through it in a grandma voice. 'There are no girl dinosaurs!' he giggled. 'Raaaaa!' Strange – not sure where baby dinosaurs come from, then.

Buying a waterproof jacket – same thing. We just want to buy a warm, waterproof jacket. Dee and me went to the shop – we picked up a purple and pink starry one (aimed at girls) and a green one (aimed at boys). Same price, same style, but different fabric. The boys' one had a rougher texture, kind of criss-crossed threads. Dee asked the assistant why and if one was more waterproof. 'No, they're the same – the green one just has ripstop fabric so it's more durable for the sort of things boys do, climbing trees and stuff.' Are you fucking serious? Where are these myths coming from? So the girls jackets, with one catch or tear, are fucked. Ripped. Done. This isn't indoor clothing, party clothing, these are warm, waterproof, outdoor jackets! I got the same thing in the shoe shop – explanation for the lack of waterproof or gripping girls' shoes given to me by a shop assistant obviously told that in training – that girls go outside less, climb less or perhaps that they like having wet bodies and feet more maybe? They like getting colds more?

We are so weird and we are passing it on to our kids. Sometimes I wish I could move into a cave away from adverts and TVs and posters and people who say things to my kid like 'Oh, do you like the train?' in an annoyingly surprised tone of voice because she's chosen to play with that toy over the doll. Today. Maybe tomorrow it'll be a different toy she picks. She likes dolls too.

Maybe the doll could drive the train, perhaps? Up your arse perhaps? Sorry, just annoyed about this today.

19 MAY

2 years 2 months

8 p.m.

Yesterday was beautiful. I spent all day in the park, in the woods, running about. I love it when kids are just kids. When they can just do what they want to do. It's also lovely to be outside, away from all computers and emails and phone calls. Away from work.

I had a dream last night. It was horrible, completely over the top. The park had been split into pink and blue. Everything painted one colour or the other. All the trees were painted blue and Little One was told she couldn't climb any of them because it wasn't for girls to get messy. My son (in my dream) was then called 'gay' for catching butterflies. I think all the 'girls'–'boys' labels are freaking me out – even in my sleep now!

Splitting Kids (Dream)

I like to go into forests and take my kids out to the park
I like to sit with them at bedtime, tell them stories, point at stars
I like doing things together that are free
where you can play and chat and run around
and not spend too much money

They say 'Mummy, can we go and play?'
We get our coats and run
but today our trusty play park wasn't so much fun.

The one gate that was there last week had now been split in two
The left-hand door was pink and the right-hand door was blue
The left-hand door said 'Girls', the right-hand door said 'Boys'
The play park had been sorted like every shop does to their toys.

The swings were on the girls' side, sprayed in pretty glitter paint
The slide was on the boys', and the wobbling bridge and train,
The fireman's pole was blue 'cos we know girls cannot slide
    down those
All they do is dance around them, twist and twirl and point
    their toes

The roundabout was with the girls, shaped into a princess's
    crown,
And a brick wall down the middle separated all the middle
    ground

The mud was on the boys' side, and the puddles and the grass,
But the sky was on the girls' side with the clouds shaped into
    hearts.
The trees were on the boys' side, 'cos the girls who climbed all
    fell
And the flowers were on the girls' side, 'cos little boys don't like
    to smell

A net was built which reached to space and a tunnel dug below
So that the park rangers could tell all the animals which side to
    go

The butterflies and birds were trapped and forced to fly on girly
    left
But the bugs and beetles underground were forced below our
    future men
The duck pond was on the left so girls could feed the little duck-
    lings
But the duck weed and the dirt were on the right with stones
    and twigs

The rain and grey-cloud thunderstorms and lightning struck the
    boys' side
'Cos girls' clothes didn't keep them warm and they didn't like
    the noises
The warm, golden sunshine and white fluffy clouds
Were told to shine for girls alone so they could smile and dance
    about

The girls were given mirrors and the boys were given swords
Blood was on the boys' side (except for period blood of course).

My son and daughter ran around, a bit confused but soon relaxed,
And any kid who tried to cross was labelled gay, tomboy or bad
And when their bellies started rumbling and hunger had kicked
    in
We came out of the play park and found a picnic spot to sit in

I got out the apples, orange squash, cheese sandwiches and rolls
I told them both a story about billy-goats and trolls
Then took out the picnic flask with one straw for each kid
But just as they put the straws up to their little thirsty lips
The park ranger was upon us selling 'official' food and drink
A picnic box of blue juice and another box of pink

'I'm afraid you cannot share those things between your girl and
        boy,'
He begged,
''Cos if we split your kids up, we sell twice as many toys,'
He said.
'We have Disney princess juice for girls and Mike the Knight
        for future kings
Branded yoghurts, branded sweets, just buy two of everything
Lego blocks to build a plane or Lego friends with flower
        stalls
Pink Kinder eggs for fannies, blue Kinder eggs for balls.'

My kids were confused at first but soon fitted right in
My daughter learnt her princess pose and my son practised
        fighting
And now every night I call my kids for bedtime one by one
I read my son a Superhero comic and my girl a book called
        Fashion Love
I kiss my daughter on the cheek and give my son a firm high-five
And we look out of the window and stare into the night
My son looks for planets, Mars of course, not Venus or the
        moon,
And my daughter looks at stars because they twinkle just like
        diamonds do.
I take them to the toilet to do their final bedtime loo
My daughter does a rainbow wee, my son a massive stinking
        poo
I tuck them into bed and pull up covers lined with trains and
        hearts
My daughter falls asleep so sweetly, my son falls asleep and
        farts

And as the sun sets on another day and the daylight turns to
    dark
I pray those toy shops never get their hands upon our forests or
    our parks.

9 p.m.

The Whole World

He had the whole world in his hands
when I was at school
He had the mountains and the rivers
the sun and the moon
He had the whole wide world
we sang it out of tune
and now she's starting the
sing-along too.

He's got the whole world
in His hands
and I have tried to read the palm-lines
like held out maps
walked across His world
the tune forever at my back
He's got the whole world
in His hands

Hands

I was always told
that Jesus' hands were charmed
One touch upon a stranger's head
and they would fall into his arms
– cured

I always thought
my own hands and palms were pretty weak
until one small touch upon your forehead
calmed you back
to sleep

I am trying hard to be open-minded, but the panic is rushing through my body quite a lot these days. I mean, I've been panicking since she was born: that I'm not doing things right; not feeding her right; not teaching her enough; not outside enough; not doing enough crafts (which, to be honest, I'm not sooo keen on) or painting or walking or anything. Every bloody thing.

But today, it's another panic, it's making my blood a little hot and my heart race a little more and I'm trying to be calm about it. But I'm slowly realising what a male-centred world my daughter is growing up in. Male, white, heterosexual. I feel like she's two years old and indoctrination is slowly seeping and creeping into her brain in a way I don't feel I can stop. I wish I could, but I don't want to bring my daughter up in a bubble, away from the local groups, school, films, books. I wouldn't want that at all. I couldn't do that anyway.

I remember a kid at school whose parents didn't let her watch any telly or listen to the radio or pop music. We went to her birthday party. There was no junk food, no music – no nothing, really. And she was bullied so badly. I remember me and my friend Jodie trying to entertain people at the party by wearing frisbees as mini-skirts and doing a joke catwalk show. I totally understand why people do this to protect their kids. But at the time, I didn't, everyone just thought she was odd. I don't know if that's fair. I really don't know. Either way, I don't have the option to do that, because Little One's not always with me anyway and I don't live in a bubble.

So I'm just getting frustrated and don't really know what to do. The way we push ideas onto our children is making me want to scream. Quietly, to myself, every night.

Example 1: Toddler Group

Today Little One asked me which man made ladybirds. I said that men didn't make ladybirds, that no one really knows how they came to exist and people believe all sorts of different things. She looked at me like I was totally stupid and repeated: 'Man made ladybirds.' She continued: 'And trees and flowers and monkeys.' On 'monkey', I realised where this was coming from. The toddler-group songs. It's in a church, and while Dee leaves before the songs at the end when *he* takes her, I've always felt like that would be rude. Most of the men leave before the end. I put it down to the fact they are more embarrassed to sing baby songs. In my head I thought: the church is opening its doors to us, the volunteers are making me hot tea, and the least I can do is not shun their songs, whatever I think of the religion itself, it's the community that counts here.

Now my head is going through all the Christian songs they sing there, slowly realising there has not been one during the entire year that I've been going that mentions anything to do with girls, women, females – He made the world, He made the animals, from the tiny, tiny ant to the huge elephant. He is great. He loves me. He made fucking everything. She loves the hand movements. They're really catchy and sweet to watch. We also sing 'The Grand Old Duke of York' each week.

I spoke about this to a friend. He gave the same reply I've been hearing for years: *Everyone knows 'He' means 'God' and therefore includes us all. It's not a human 'He'.* Just like 'mankind' actually means 'humankind' and 'guys' can mean 'women and men'. The thing is, though, for me as a female, it doesn't. 'He' means 'he'. For me, and obviously I see now, for my two-year-old daughter.

I don't understand how people keep on with this concept. If it was flipped the other way round and we referred to God as 'She', to humans as 'womankind', to a group of men as 'hey girls', in no way would men feel included in the use of those words. It's stupid to think that they would. It's stupid to think it doesn't have an effect on us fannies.

So my daughter thinks that a mortal man invented everything she loves on this planet. I can talk to her about it as much as I like, but the songs seem to be more powerful. Don't stay for the songs next time. Don't worry about offending people so much. It's OK to have a different belief in ladybird creation and still be friends with those who are more passionate about the song lyrics than you. And the women who run it are so damn kind.

Example 2: Toys

I'm slowly realising that the default for any toy or children's character is male. And I'm not exaggerating here: I know there are mummy and daddy bear stories and female animals in books and on television, but in general, if an animal just looks like an animal, my daughter, and every other kid I play with, assumes it's a male. A man or a boy. A plain teddy bear, a dinosaur toy, a dog, a giraffe – it doesn't matter what the graphic or the toy – it's a man. In order for it to become female the characters are given bows or a hairband or a dress or, more frequently, eyelashes. Long eyelashes to distinguish them from the men. Think Mickey and Minnie. *Peppa Pig* is an exception though: Dad has a goatee and Mum has eyelashes. Most of the time the male animal is just an animal and the female is an animal *plus a feature*. The default is male. If I suggest to Little One that her teddy is a girl, she disagrees, unless she puts a hairband on it. With real animals it depends. She was shocked that there were female dogs. Equally though, that there were male rabbits or butterflies. Confused kids!

Example 3: Books

This is a big one for me. I read a lot. I love reading. It's one of my favourite things to do in life and with Little One now as well. We go to the library once a week and get five books out and it's one of the best trips we have. I used to let her pick her books. Free choice, not a pushy parent. Go crazy, love.

Till I realised a few things about a lot of the books. Firstly, most of the characters are white. So my curly-haired, brown-skinned daughter rarely, if ever, got a chance to read books where anyone looked in any way like her because, statistically, she'd likely not find one. Secondly, like toys, most of the books these days are split into girls' and boys' books. There are not that many that have a mix of boys and girls playing together. So she rarely read books with little boys in. Thirdly, there are absolutely no gay people in any of the books I ever saw. None. It doesn't exist – but there are a lot of couples and love stories.

Trying to level this a bit has been bloody eye-opening at times. As Little One plays on the train in the library and looks at books I flick through the shelves, mainly thinking: *Boys and girls, brown skin*. Especially having a main character with brown skin, not just a token mate on one page of a story or a patronising factual kids book about 'children in Africa'. A few authors have been superstars in this; Rachel Isadora, Eileen Browne and Gill Lobel are our moment's favourites. My family are on board and everyone understands why we might want to balance out the pallor of the book collection. They understand for the same reason why I scouted high and low to find Barbies with different skin tones, after Little One was given, and loves playing with, three blondes. I used to play with Barbies. Non-white Barbies are more expensive. But I bought three the same week I finished Toni Morrison's *The Bluest Eye* and Little One kept insisting she had blue eyes like me until I played Van Morrison on loop.

So most people seem to agree this is important. But moving on to sexuality is another matter entirely. That is not OK. That has elicited other reactions from people around me. I kind of expected them, but it's still quite amazing to see. Of all the books people have given us, I'd say about 40 per cent have a couple in them, always straight and always married. A lot of the stories centre on the marriage – fairytales obviously, but more modern ones as well. Marriage, marriage, straight, straight, straight. Fine.

The thing I found interesting, though, was the reaction when I ordered a book called *King and King* by Linda de Haan and Stern Nijland. I wanted to see what Little One's reaction would be to this book, where two princes marry. I had it delivered, read it to her one night, she smiled and said 'Lovely', then picked up the next book. So a two-year-old was fine with that. Not a shit was given. Other people, however, adults I mean, seemed pretty worried by it.

As well as just rolling eyes and laughing, comments included:

Are you trying to make her gay?

I know you want her to be a lesbian.

What point are you trying to make?

I don't think this is appropriate.

But mainly it was suggested that I was trying to somehow push Little One into being gay. Indoctrinate her. Force her kicking and screaming into lesbianism (despite it being about two gay men) against her will by reading her one book about this fact of human nature – that not all people are straight. I now have one book, among about a hundred we read, with a gay couple in it. No one, absolutely no one, suggested that maybe the million books, films, cartoons featuring straight couples and marriage could possibly be indoctrinating her in a way similar to what they were suggesting for 'gayness'.

I've had the same angry reaction about the Christian songs too. I started singing 'he and she' instead of 'He' at one point. I also changed 'He's got the whole world in his hands' to 'They've got the whole world in their hands'; and whenever I do this I always have people telling me I'm 'over the top', 'making a fuss', 'being stupid'. An annoying, moany, miserable slag of a woman. Same reaction I get online to poems about being female. Slag. Prude. Ugly. Bitch. Need more cock in your life.

I find really angry reactions to anything that rocks the boat a bit. And an absolute refusal by those people to consider that singing a multitude of songs about 'He' being brilliant and 'He' being the saviour of the universe might possibly leave a tiny dent in a kid's thinking. They just see any argument against it as being anti men. Rather than anti little girls growing up with a sense that women do fuck all, and little boys growing up with a sense of failure if they do not become God-like superheroes.

So I can't talk about women, and I can't talk about gay people. 'Cos that's indoctrination and it just makes me a pain in the arse. A few people – way fewer, though – have said the same about me being a bit on guard to make sure there are some non-Caucasian characters at some point in Little One's life. Those people, all Caucasian, seem unable to come to terms with the idea that if they grew up only seeing – I don't know – Somalian-, Kenyan-, Korean-, Iranian-, Syrian-featured people in books, birthday cards, comics, films, TV shows etc. they might be affected by it in some way. Trying to buy a birthday card for Dee's family possibly opened up my eyes to this the most. 'Yeah,' Dee said, 'you only get white people on these things. I just got white kids on all my birthday cards growing up. And my toys. And books.' Slowly changing, but slowly.

I *am* on guard. And I think it's important. Because indoctrination seems to be seeping in, and my trying to do whatever I can to prevent that makes people strangely angry at me. I think I'd prefer this, though, than my daughter continuing to think during the most important early years of her life that a straight, Caucasian man is inventing ladybirds the world over.

This does not mean I'm anti straight Caucasian males or don't understand the particular traumas the white male may experience. It's about the basics of a child's understanding of the world and her place in it.

This stuff is much harder than feeding a small baby.

2 years 2 months

9 p.m.

At The Door

Stand back. Back off. Breathe out –
You're almost out the door now.
Be there. to help. if asked –
She's only two years old now.
She wants. to try. herself –
So let your arms drop down now.
Stand back. Back off. Breathe out –
There's no point getting stressed now.
She's almost. done. her buttons –
It doesn't matter some are wrong now.
If you. hurry her. she'll panic –
Her shoes are almost on now.
The left. is on. the right –
But no need to step in yet.
She's already looking down now –
Now she's. trying out. the left.
Don't let. your blood. get hot.

Don't let. your patience. blow.
Relax. Breathe out. Be proud.
She's only two years old.

Last week, I had to fight a very strong urge to ditch work, go to the pub and scream into a pint for three hours. Sometimes getting a toddler ready is like that. Sometimes it is totally fine. Sometimes it is an utter joy to watch little fingers scrabble to button jackets wonkily and push shoes on the wrong feet and then stand up, proud as a peacock, to display their talent. Sometimes it is hard not to move their fingers aside and do it much more quickly for them. Let her do it, Dee will remind me. Let her do it, I'll remind him. Teamwork.

Little One wants to do everything herself now. It is a beautiful thing. But everything takes a tad longer because of that. It is hard to be patient sometimes. I want her to learn life skills – dressing herself, tying her shoes, getting her bag ready – I really do. But Lord God, sometimes it takes so long to get ready! Sometimes it takes gritted teeth, deep breaths and the constant thought that it is OK to be late, she is learning, she is learning. Resist. the. urge. to. help. her.

People often say that parents or carers who 'leave employment' in order to raise their kids are losing valuable skills and CV points and job training.

Personally, the task of managing to get my toddler ready as she breaks down in tears (because she could not work out which way her pants go on), goes into a strop (because I tried to help), slams her door, hides in her bed in protest, then takes an hour to brush her teeth, and out of the door without losing my temper, raising my hand, crying hysterically or throwing myself on the kitchen floor – is a miracle. And we were still only a bit late in dropping her off at Grandma's. To me, that's a skill and should definitely be seen credibly on any CV.

I think that after that morning I finally felt finally ready to apply for the job of chief ambassador of the UN peacekeeping conflict resolution force. As stated in Article 1 of the UN Charter, the UN is expected 'to maintain international peace and security ... to take effective collective measures for the prevention and removal of threats to peace ... and to bring about by peaceful means ... adjustment or settlement of international disputes'.

Now, I went to what I think is a good school – St Bart's Comprehensive, Newbury. I worked geekily hard and with a lot of help from family and teachers and the fact I had my own bedroom to work in, got into Cambridge University to study languages. After I graduated, I then worked in a nightclub and a shop to pay for a part-time MSc in Development Studies with Economics at the School of Oriental and African Studies in London. I read lots of papers and studies about international conflict. I wanted to work in that area somehow.

None of those qualifications – plus that fact that I still could not afford to do a free internship with any charity after graduating – made me feel capable of applying for the kind of job I wanted. I was always sure I wasn't good enough, no matter how hard I worked. My supervisor at Cambridge used to call it the 'state-school mentality'. But doing the morning drop-off day after day without losing my temper, I finally feel ready. In fact, I feel that the new skills I have now acquired as a parent should be a mandatory part of any application for a UN or government position requiring any sort of negotiation or discussion skills. Instead of unaffordable internship placements for extremely well-off graduates (no grudge here), I now imagine an interview might go something a bit more like this:

Hello, please come in. Which position are you applying for?

Er, Head of the UN peacekeeping mission.

And why do you feel qualified for this job?

Well, I graduated from Eton and have a first-class degree in politics from Oxford University, a PhD in conflict resolution and international peacekeeping and I have been on an unpaid internship for an international charity for the last three years, as well as having experience in my father's department of the World Bank from the age of three.

OK, fine. Are you a parent or guardian of a child?

Erm, no. I don't have kids.

Have you ever spent at least three full days and nights as the sole carer of a child or other person in need?

Er, what? No.

Have you ever had a baby's poo spurt up your arms while changing a nappy and still carried on saying 'Googoo' and smiling as they wee in your face?

Er, no.

Have you ever had to get a child dressed and out of the house, been able to keep your cool and react calmly and peaceably under the intense pressure of tantrums and crying and screams and then stand on the pavement as other people walk past you, smiling at them red-faced whilst your child lies on the floor screaming 'Go away, I'm never speaking to you again!' and refuses to move – without crying or screaming yourself?

Er, no.

Have you ever had to settle a dispute with a child or group of children without resorting to fist-banging, shouting 'Ra ra, Mr Speaker', raising your voice or laughing in a pompous, arrogant manner at them?

Er, no.

OK, thank you. We'll let you know. We were really looking for someone who has toddler-care skills. Primary teaching might work too. We'll call you.

II

SUMMER
TWO YEARS THREE MONTHS
GRATEFUL

2 years 3 months

1 a.m.

It is a beautiful, sunny day. Our friends Louise and Steve have had a second baby. Premature again, and they are not sure she will survive. I cannot imagine that and I don't know what to do to help, if there's anything I *can* do. She is waiting to kiss her baby, that's all she wants to do this week, just a kiss with her baby. I promise myself to savour this summer, every minute, every kiss and walk and cry. I sent Louise this poem, no idea if I should have and now I'm a bit worried I overstepped the mark. I don't know how they feel at all. It's just when I write a poem based on someone else I always feel it belongs more to them than to me. I hope she doesn't mind me writing it. I hug Little One while she's sleeping. I sleep on the floor in her room for some reason. I can't leave her tonight. I can't sleep. I just stare at her face, my palm on her chest every five minutes checking the breaths are still strong enough to dream through.

Small Gold

She's almost the size of an outstretched palm
With tubes through her airways and lungs

365

A bud so curious she opened her petals
Before they were quite ready for sun

And her mum sits beside her like a guardian angel
Every morning she wakes, every night
Protecting her body by giving up hers
Filling her belly just right

With foods she should have so her milk might be golden
As hours she can sleep are rightfully stolen
Waking in dreams and napping for seconds
As days sail away into baby's protection

As family balance baby and beautiful child
Whose jokes and laughter inspire them to smile
A beam of a toddler-like sunlight and laughter
Reminding you what will come after

Family tight, two girls, mum and dad
As life ticks along in slow-motion drags
Holding each other up through more sleepless naps
As the world still turns as it had

So if you want to know true love
Stop watching films
Full of glamorous couples and Hollywood stills
Kissing in rain in beautiful clothes
Wrapped in their arms like the whole world should know
'Cos if you don't know true love
This is it
In eyes so tired they're in constant half-lids
Closed and opened at each cry she makes

To a close woman's body forever awake
Taking the time of your life for another
Between newly met sister and father and mother
It is sunrise to sunset in quickened-beat hearts
And minds frozen in time every time you're apart

So if you want to know true love, this is it
Watching a baby, for days, just waiting to kiss
And if there's a reason why we're here, on this planet, this is it
To realise the love we have to give

So if you want to know true love
You might find it in this seed
A little bud who bloomed ahead
So curious to see
And though she might be as tiny as her father's longing hold
She already knows a love
So pure it tastes like gold.

Louise messaged me this morning and said thanks for the poem. I am so relieved. She's still at the hospital. I read an article today about Brazil's milk banks, especially aimed at saving premature babies. They have the highest breastmilk donation in the world. The fire service – firefighters – run the collections under their 'saving lives' remit. It's annoying that I'm starting to understand the absolute magic of this milk stuff now, but felt weird when I had it in my own body. I should've donated. I didn't even know it was a thing.

Anyway, her baby is stable. How anyone deals with this stuff is beyond me. I am taking Little One to the park again.

19 JULY

2 years 4 months

2 a.m.

I had a gig in Norwich last week. It finished at midnight and I had to walk to the car park and drive home alone. I had threats online from a guy who said he was getting a group together – said he was affiliated to the EDL – to come to my gig and show me 'how much they appreciated my ideas about immigration'. All posted below my YouTube videos. My friend said if I didn't go I'd be giving in to them. Easy for him to say, huh, when he's not the one worrying he might be followed to the car park after the gig and beaten to shit.

I went to the gig and nothing happened, apart from me being a nervous wreck. On the way home I was caught in the most torrential storm I've ever known. I couldn't see through the windscreen and I couldn't stop anywhere. I was in tears the whole drive home. I am so tired of juggling parenthood and gigs and my day job, and I'm bored with online trolls threatening me and telling me I do nothing but write poems and fanny about when the truth is I hardly have time to wipe my arse. Sometimes I wish I could be at home every day, go to the park and sleep more. No, that's not true. I just wish I could sleep more.

Rainstorm

The car radio spoke of warfare on the news
The rain in front poured down

Windscreen wipers frantic spray
to clear the clouds in squeaking sounds

I've never really worried about dying before
through rain pumped down to pavement roads

and when the car lost control
for the fourth time tonight
and as the lightning above
sparked up the sky
on a drowned-out motorway night
I started panicking
for home

I always imagined that if I were dying
I'd be desperate to travel the world

trek Machu Picchu before it's too late
I imagined some secret donation hurled at me

I imagined I'd want to do all that I could before
death took me down

but drowning in rain
mistaking clutch push for brakes
my hands grasping the steering wheel
to straighten the shakes

the fall of the tree as lightning axed down
I imagined the sound it would make as it hit

each lorry I passed I was sure that was it
and every time I thought about this

I wanted desperately just to get home

To see her asleep
to see him asleep
to feel their warm skin
and hold their soft cheeks
there were no panic-led dreams
of the places not been to
just thoughts of the two of you
and wanting to be with you
panic to get near to you
one great last time

and I realised if I had one more minute of life
I wouldn't want to be travelling or hitching a skydive

no bucket-list dreams, not any of that
I would want to be sitting inside our small flat

holding her close to me, us all
silently sat
in a smile

2 years 5 months

Falling in Love

I was sick last night. Food poisoning or bug or something. Dee was away working. I started feeling real queasy at one a.m. just as you woke up crying. I took you into bed and tried to get you back to sleep but I needed to vomit. I said quietly, 'I need to go to the bathroom, Mummy feels sick.' You followed me, sat behind me on the dark floor and rubbed my back. Then refused to leave the bathroom for the next three hours, got your blankets and camped out with a few plastic fish and a vomiting mum.

I fell in love again last night.

2 years 5 months

Rain on Our Faces

I'm the luckiest person alive
with my kid by my side
and the sun in the sky
fruit on the trees
and bees buzzing by
they whisper the meaning of life if you listen

In my own little kitchen
Little One sitting
crumbling butter
flour in fingers
covered in sugar
and a bag full of blackberries
picked by the road

My kid's cheeks are gleaming
and the smell of the crumble cooking
overwhelms my tired eyes

I am the luckiest person alive.

Picking strawberries
by the wall in the city
finding pear trees and figs
if you look very closely
as the juices cover her entire face
and we pray for the Autumn
for the apples to taste

Walking round streets
on the days I'm still there
spying for fruit trees
or bushes with her

I'm the luckiest mum in the world.

So when you tell me our flat is too small again
I don't care
and no, we don't own our very own garden
we share.
but we're safe and we're healthy and each day that's still there

I am the happiest person alive.

I want to smother her skin
in keylock kisses
protect her from the world beyond
flowers and bushes
climbing trees in the park
taking walks after dark
I'm completely in love

the forests don't scare me
society does

and I'm trying to give her some space to unglove
before she's packed up and picked on
and packaged and airbrushed
before the boys are told blue and the girls are told pink
and she's told what to learn and told how to think
with posters of princesses, white-blonde and thin
and she wonders why none of those match her reflection

So I'll stay in the park where the playing is free
and there's no separation with pink and blue trees
and we'll pick fruit and eat it as much as we can
while she builds up her strength to sail on dry land
by herself.

But we're happy and healthy and each day that remains
I will be grateful for each drop of rain

as we run under trees
and shelter
till sun comes again.

2 years 5 months

Today was bliss. Little One is currently obsessed with her cardboard-box fridge and oven and now when I cook, she always asks for ingredients for her pan. She keeps telling me she's cooking soup and I realise we do have that about four days a week. I'm turning into my gran: 'Soup and pudding all week for tea and then a Sunday lunch,' she always used to tell me. So Little One sits and stirs her soup. I've noticed that whatever she makes, she eats; it's jokes. It looks gross. I gave her a few peas, a bit of cheese, beetroot, pasta shells and a carrot. She added hot water, stirred it all then drank it when it was cool enough. All of it, big lumps of soggy cheese floating on watery pink soup. Half-cooked pasta. But she made it, I guess that's the most exciting part. I'm loving this age.

I love cooking with her. I try so hard not to keep stopping her as she gets the kitchen covered in flour. *Just let her try, Hollie, stop butting in!* Not sure I'm ready to be a mother still, but it's pretty fascinating right now. I just hope she's enjoying it too. She's smiling at least. Phew.

Nicking Strawberries

I want to cook for you
my baby
that is all I want to do now

You've had your milk, you're good for more
I want to teach you how to climb up trees
and mash your apple stew now

I want to cook for you
I want to chop the veg and wash the fruit
and watch you as you giggle
above a chin that kisses fresh pear juice.

I want to cook for you
my Little One
chopped onions, garlic, rosemary
plump tomatoes
pot lid on and watch you as you chat with me

I want to cook you rainbows
watch you grow
and see you find that pot of gold
in blackberries picked down the street
and strawberries nicked from city walls.

I want to cook for you
as you grow tall
I want to feed your heartbeats
feed it all
our kitchen and our wallets small
but cookbook pages free for all

I want to cook for you
and watch you
with bread bombs thrown in carrot soups
feed you from your head to roots

as beetroot paints your tongue bright pink
and you stick it out at me in pride
I watch your frown lines come as spices sing
I want to feed your childhood cravings
with all the perfect things

and now I see you sitting
in the kitchen
telling me you're 'on the cooking'
wooden spoons
a little pan
banging lids
like only kids can
a cardboard box
your fridge and oven
sitting peeling paper onions
asking me for scraps of cheese
making up new recipes

You're tipping cinnamon on carrot slices
bread and milk and peanut butter

You giggle that you're making supper
and I'm hoping it all tastes as nice
as the life you give me
by your side
watching as your eyes grow big
at first new sips
and dips in sauces.

I want to cook you
all the finest courses

my knowledge can afford
so you can run like wind through fields of mud
splash in puddles
climb up trees

I want to cook you all the energy your lovely muscles need
to write and read
jump and breathe
to hear and see
so eat with me
I learnt for you
it's something that I could not do before
and it makes my heartbeat lighten if I hear you ask for more

And yes sometimes the food goes on the floor
on the floor where you sit stirring pans
so sit with me and hold my hand
Messy clothes?
I don't give a damn
I'm trying to dress your insides right
so beautifully clean
I want to feed your every heartbeat
so they can keep up with your dreams

I'm travelling this world in cookbooks
I care what you eat, not if you look good
so bang your pots and fill your pans

I'm trying to cook you
the best start in life
I can.

12

AUTUMN
TWO YEARS SIX MONTHS
BARBED-WIRE BODIES

Barbed Wire

You

Marks out of Ten

Megatron

2 years 5 months

In a shop today, Little One screamed to Dee, who was stood at the tills, 'I love you, Daddy', over and over again. Dee's face was brightly blushed, everyone was staring at him. I love kids. I especially love it when she embarrasses him like this. Only kids have the ability to bring that out in people, I think. I tell her I don't think he heard and to shout it again. He's cringing at the counter.

When do we stop being so honest? So open with our feelings? It's so cool to see what we'd be like without all the 'teaching' we get. Dee – he's always so cool and collected. Moments like this are gold. It's embarrassing when she shouts 'Is that man pregnant?' or 'Are you doing a poo?' in public toilets. But this show of open, honest emotion was great.

Barbed Wire

Dee says his compliments are wrapped in barbed wire
'Cos he's gotta be a man
He jokes he's gotta be a man
And he will walk with me by shining streams

But he will not hold my hand
No he will not hold my hand

And he tells me that he thinks I'm great
Then breaks into a sweat
A red-faced fumbled wreck
As he covers compliments in buts and ifs in
Reels of barbed-wire fences
Help to harden senses

And it takes me back to days at school
When the boys would pull my hair
Then ask me on a date
And we would walk around the netball court
Hand in shaking hand
Gums cut by my three-year brace
Getting older awkward silent moments

The shit never changed
Nothing's ever changed

Feelings that we want to share
But barbed wire's in the way
Barbed wire's in the way.

The first time he said the words
Lying face to face
Throat dry face to face
I love you felt like letting loose

That shit's so hard to say
It took so long to say.
'Cos we're so used to covering and jokes
That real talk is so hard
Heartbeats pound so fast

He says he was brought up taught to be a bloke
Feelings bottled up
And his barbed wire gave him cuts

And though I've taken out some of the knots
And he isn't quite so sharp
A slowly softened heart

But when I saw his eyes with heavy sobs
As he held her in his arms
A baby in his arms
I can feel the heat she brings him
As she covers him in hugs
I can almost see the metal melting
No holds back showing love

She says, 'I love you so much, Daddy'
She kisses off his face
No embarrassment to tell
Nearly fifty times a day

Each time my heartbeat breaks
With her he lets his feelings shine
'Cos kids don't hold their feelings back

I think we could learn a lot
from what they do and what they say

No barbed wire in the way
No barbed wire in the way.

3 SEPTEMBER

2 years 5 months

I took Little One swimming today. I love how warm the kids' pool is. My mate says it's wee but I'm not sure I care. So we went swimming. I had promised all week. Then yesterday I came on. I don't mind deep-water swimming on my period, but when you're crawling around at knee level in a toddlers pool in a swimsuit it's a bit more awkward. But I'd promised. I've always been open about periods. My gran tells me she wasn't allowed to talk about them at all and I know there is still a massive amount of shaming and global traumas about the fact that females start bleeding once a month at puberty. So I don't want her to see it in any way as a shameful, awful, embarrassing thing. I also don't really get how anyone does manage to hide this stuff from their kids, 'cos mine doesn't even let me wee in peace and we're only one loo.

She doesn't bat an eyelid now. In fact, she now insists on unwrapping sanitary pads for me like presents. Last week, I went to my friend Steph's house and found that Little One and her son had rummaged our bags and stuck a sanitary towel to each of their heads, as they came pegging past us.

So we get to the pool changing room and I realise I forgot to put in a tampon at home. I'm not sure about showing her those yet, purely 'cos I'm worried she'll try to copy me. So we're in the changing room and I ask her to look in my bag to get something while I try a lightning manoeuvre. It doesn't work. Blood on my thighs and fingers. She turns back and gasps. We go to the showers so I can wash it off and I try again. It works but by now she has five million questions about it all. I answer them and tell her I get worried sometimes about leaking.

We walk to the pool – she refuses to hold my hand to the pool 'because blood mummy'. I washed it off but still, she's having none of it!

I then sit in the pool as she swims about me. After five minutes, she darts under the water in her goggles beside me and when she's up for air, tells me loudly 'don't worry, no blood'. Thanks, I say. She plays this game for the next hour, my face a bloody crimson.

Sometimes this openness has its drawbacks.

Nearly 2 years 6 months

Today Little One touched my belly. Sweet. Then kissed it. Sweet. Poked it, pushed it, grabbed it and patted it. Sweet. Then said she loved it cos it was like Play-Doh – 'and I love Play-Doh, Mum!' 'Thanks', I smiled, through gritted – I am trying so hard not to pass on any body insecurities to you at all – teeth. I grabbed it and played with it too, criticising each poke in my head, loving it out loud to her. I want to love it in my head too. I really, really want to see my own skin the way she sees it right now.

You

You are the reason why
my belly tripled in size
and left striped lines
across my skin when you left

You are the reason why my chest moved
from an A cup to a C
to a double E
and back again
to keep you well fed

You are the reason why
my old-size jeans
no longer fit me
why the belt
no longer reaches the stretch
of my slightly wider hips

You are the reason I miss sleep
Why my eyelids feel weak

You are the reason why my heart
skips a beat
every night
Why my laughter lines double
and grow deeper
each day

You are the smile carved
like a permanent mark
on my face
Every time you wake me up
at six a.m. to play
Drumming on my belly
Blowing raspberries on my skin
and I joke that one day I might put you back in
and when I tell you that you lived there
you tell me it's a fib
asking me for proof
like a toddler detective

I point to the place
you lift my top up a little

then bang on my stretch marks
and giggle.

Marks out of Ten

I've got marks on my face to match my age.
I've got a mark on my forehead where a chickenpock remained.
I've got a mark on my back from my roller-skating days.
You might like to take a look at them one day.

I've got marks on my cheeks from where I slept.
I've got marks on my stomach where it shrank after it stretched.
I've got marks on my breasts. The baby was well fed.
I've got marks, like everybody else.

I've got a mark on my ear where my bike chains fell and shook.
I've got a mark on my hand from a pan I loved to cook with.
I've got marks on my nails from the bites I always took.
I've got marks. You can read me like a book.

I've got marks on my feet from all the places that I've stood.
I've got marks beside my eyes from smiles and feeling good.
I've got marks around my lips from laughing till I shook.
Twelve marks out of ten.
That's pretty good.

2 years 6 months

Me and Dee went to see the new *Transformers* film. Megatron versus Optimus Prime. I got annoyed about everyone banging on about how cool Transformers were. I wrote this poem and read it to Dee. He said it was the worst poem and it goes totally downhill after I stop talking about Transformers! 'Seriously, Hollie, you need more Transformers in there. Less women, more Transformers!' ...

Megatron

He said: 'Megatron's the best one
If I was one, it's him.
Optimus Prime's all nice and stuff
But it's Megatron who really wins.'

I've listened so many times to this
Since last week's sodding *Transformers* hit
And I smile until today I say
'Megatron ain't shit
Last year my hip bones moved
Another half an inch
Back together.'

He said, 'Hollie, Megatron lives for ever.'
I said, 'Megatron's not real
If you wanna hold a real live transformer
Come and have a feel.'
And I pushed his fingers closer
And then right inside my stomach
To feel the gap my muscles left
From something I now know a bit
as birth

And I knew that this would hurt
But I did not know the rest
That there'd be a hole inside my stomach
till the day I'm laid to rest

'And no, you're right,' I said
'It's not the same
I didn't turn into a car
I turned into a factory
A life support and
Cooker

As my body started morphing
My insides realigned
My digestive system shifted
And completely redesigned itself.
No help from the Decepticons or the Autobots

What vitamins I'd got moved from my blood into hers now
The direction of my nutrients redirected into her
How?
I don't know

Everyone sees the stomach grow
We do not see the rest
Ribcage cranking up
To make more space for baby's legs
Diaphragm moves down
My womb filled up with fluid
And a brown line on your skin appears
And no one even drew it
A brown line on my skin
From between my legs to boobs
The only line a child can see
To lead them to the food
Labour came and went
Something that I won't forget
Baby now in my arms
And my system shifted once again
Digestion redirected to
Two breasts that grew one night
Bigger than a large ripe pair of cantaloupes
'Get me a pump!' I screamed
Genuinely worried that they might explode
My boobs stay warm to heat the milk
My nipples make a hole
And every time the baby drinks
The suction
Makes
My
Womb shrink back
My hips move back
My ribs and diaphragm move back
My hair grow back
My back stretch back

And after two more years of doing that
My system shifted back
Nutrients shot back into my own body's blood again

And now I'm nearly back to how I was
Before that seed took life
Complete transformation
without one single robot fight
But no one
makes an action film of this!

In fact all my body has to show for it
Are the markings on my belly
My hips bones stayed a bit apart
And my boobs are pretty saggy
But the saddest thing of all
Is I'm told these marks are bad
But they're the only few reminders
of this process we all have
As the real lifetime transformers
I'm saying Megatron ain't shit
Compared to female bodies
To prepare to grow and feed a kid

And the only thing our body's given
For this Optimus of Primes
Is a pot of soddin' stretch-mark cream
To try to hide the signs.

2 years 6 months

I'm in Riga, in Latvia, doing a workshop and poetry slam with the British Council. A week away from home. An actual week away. In another country. With other people who don't know I'm a mum.

The first day here I did a workshop with a group of adults. Made them eat strawberries and whisper poems to each other. Yesterday, I went to the Latvia Poetry Slam, then stayed out until about four a.m. Because I can. Because I can stay out and go out raving and not come home because I do not have to get up this morning and can actually have a hangover. I can have, and recover from, a late night and a hangover. I have to give a talk at six p.m. No problem. I'm in bed till then.

It is liberating being here. I miss home. I think. No, I don't. If I'm absolutely honest with myself, I don't. I love talking to Little One on the phone because I know she's fine. I know Dee loves it too, getting me out of their hair, being able to do things his way for a week.

And really, this is amazing. It is odd. People don't know I have a child here. In fact, most of them assume I don't and have been shocked when I do a mum poem on stage. It's been so nice. They've asked me actual questions about my actual job, passions, loves. Nothing to do with motherhood. Like they actually want to know my thoughts about other things. Or just want to dance and have a laugh. I love dancing. I love dancing in big warehouses full of people I don't know and foreign voices and alcohol I've not tried. I feel like me again. Hollie. Not mum. Or girlfriend. Just Hollie. That's all these people here know.

And the bed is delicious, even with a headache and the possibility of vomiting in about ten minutes' time.

2 years 6 months

Today was a shock. Today I realised that I've been writing down things about parenthood and not always actually talking to Dee about them all. I asked if everything was OK while I was away and he said 'Yeah, cool', then looked totally sheepish.

'Really?' I asked again.

'Well, yeah,' he said.

'What was wrong?' I said.

He didn't want to tell me. Didn't want to put me off going away again. Didn't want me to feel anything about taking gigs away. I started to get worried.

'Tell me, Dee. I'll still go away.'

I don't know what I was expecting him to say, but his face was serious. Really serious. Then he told the story:

'Well, we were at a café having a meal—'

'Right.'

'And everything was fine.'

'Right.'

'And then she flipped.'

'Right.'

'She poured her whole glass of water into the spaghetti—'

'OK—'

'And I had to leave 'cos she was misbehaving.'

OK. I expected more. Sounded like a normal bad moment.

'And then what?' I said.

'Well, I just felt horrible and everyone was looking at me and I felt like it was because I was a man and they thought I couldn't look after my own kid. It was shit. I felt so angry and pissed off and I don't want to feel angry at a kid but I felt like chucking the water over her.'

'Yeah,' I said, 'I know what you mean. Sounds shit.'

He looked kind of shocked. I wasn't sure why.

'What is it?'

'Well, I just feel like you won't go away now.'

'Why not? That stuff happens to me too.'

He looked shocked again.

'No, it doesn't. You're always so calm and collected and you never get angry or think things like that. You're so fucking calm.'

To be honest, I almost spat out my tea. After nearly three years having a child together I realised that Dee genuinely thought I didn't get angry. That I didn't ever feel like pouring water over Little One or screaming or shouting at her or throwing things or dragging her out of restaurants because I was so fucking embarrassed at everyone staring at me. He didn't realise I felt like I wanted to run away, far away, when she did things like this.

'Dee! What are you on about? I feel like that loads!'

He gave me the look I gave my mum once, when I was pregnant. My mum, the calmest woman I have ever known, who never raised her fist or hand or voice at me growing up but who said, just before Little One was born: 'If you ever get to the stage you feel you might harm your child, leave it crying and leave the room. Take time out. Stand away, breathe and calm yourself down.'

'What are you on about, Mum?!' I'd said, shocked.

'I'm just saying, Hollie. You will be tired and sometimes you won't know what to do and the baby will scream and cry and you'll be drained and ... just step away and take five.'

I thought she was tripping. Until Little One was six weeks old and

I'd not slept for about five of those and she spent a full day screaming and crying and not sleeping and I was crying and pacing with her to get her to sleep and I started sobbing loudly, asking her why the hell she wasn't sleeping and then … I put her down and sat down for five minutes to remind myself it is not a baby's fault they do not sleep or stop crying. It was a good time out.

I told Dee about my mum's advice.

'What? But you never seem angry with her,' he said.

'That doesn't mean I'm not, in my head.'

So I've been writing and writing and locking away these thoughts. Dee and me do talk, we talk about everything. I thought. Or maybe we talk up to a point, and then he bottles the rest and I write the rest down. I also realised today that as a man, he has next to bugger-all of a support network to talk to. That his mates don't talk about it, worried how they'll be judged as angry thinkers; and that, unlike me, he doesn't get many 'play dates', mainly because he is male and the women seem way more wary of inviting a dad rather than a mum round their house with the kids. Which is totally and utterly shit. Him feeling like he is the only parent that ever gets raging with a child is totally shit – like even *thinking* that is an awful, awful thing, that no one around him, me included, had or would ever do. I cannot imagine how hard that must have been. I thought my anger and frustration were pretty obvious. But maybe not. Maybe I've been talking to sheets of paper and toddler-group mums and friends more than to him.

I feel terrible. How hard must it be for a lot of men looking after kids. Less support and way more fear about sharing these things. Especially those about anger and rage (which are seen as more violent in men) and sadness or tears (seen as inappropriate for men). And probably fewer friends to chat to. Unless you live in some liberal city areas where the ratio of men to women who go to these groups is more equal.

Poor guy. He had been kicking himself for days about the fact he was angry enough to want to throw water at his child, but didn't, and instead left the restaurant and went home. He's a fucking brilliant father.

'Then what happened?' I asked.

'Nothing. She was fine at home.'

I smiled at him. I feel really bad, though. That's tough. I just thought that by now everyone knew that everyone else finds this hard a lot of the time.

13

WINTER
TWO YEARS NINE MONTHS
INDEPENDENT WOMEN

2 years 8 months

I've been on the train a lot with Little One recently and I struggle to understand humans when I do. I wish I didn't have to get the train so much. My family are mainly in Scotland. My parents are near Reading, and trains are the best way to get to them with her. Booked in advance, I love getting the train. Way better than buses or cars for a kid, I think. Except those times when it is awful and I feel like I'm going to kill someone.

I went home to visit my parents. I have to get the Underground from King's Cross to the connecting train at Paddington to Newbury, as always. I have a pram, a kid, a suitcase, a bag of picnic food and a few little toys. I get to Paddington Underground and there's no working lift. I stand at the bottom of the stairs. Sometimes people help. But not always. And when they don't, it makes me want to stand and scream 'Can none of you see me? Please just give me a fucking hand,' at the top of my lungs. But instead, I feel tiny and in the way and full of zero confidence to even mutter 'Please can you help me' in mouse whispers. Last month I stood for nearly ten minutes as passengers rushed past me in their busy London way. So fucking important. No one helped. I had to leave the pram and suitcase at the bottom of the stairs and walk Little One to the top through crowds of people. I tell her to stand still at the top of the stairs – 'Please stand still Little One, you understand, do not move' – while I run back down to lug the pram and suitcase and food bag up, gripped by heart-spasming nightmares that she'll get pushed over or suddenly run off and I'll never find her again. People shoved their self-important arses past me up the stairs as I hauled it all, step by step, towards her beautiful, staring little face. I walked to the train holding her hand with tears in my eyes. I'm tired.

When I got to my parents', I felt like punching my dad. It wasn't his fault, I know. But he has a car, more free time than us, no job and no little kids. He's not obliged to visit, although I bloody love seeing him. And he says he wants to see us so I make the effort. I just wish I could film my journey and make him understand it is definitely harder for me to get to him than vice versa. I bite my lip. I want her to see her granddad and soon she'll be out of the pram and it'll be better. And we always have a great time there with my mum and dad. I just wish he understood the effect that this journey has upon my heart, soul, backbone and mental state.

The month before that, I'm on the train to Scotland to get to a gig in Edinburgh. It is a six-hour journey and I take Little One so she can visit the family while I do the gig. Six hours. For a kid that's a long time. I have a picnic packed, I make a million games out of the old cup and stirrer my tea was in. A rocket. A house. A bath. A swimming pool. Then, at some point, obviously, she wants to walk. And the train is full. I tell her to do it quietly, but she wants to talk to people. One man hides behind his paper and blanks her. She gets a little loud, so I bring her back to the seat. Others smile and it mends my heart a bit.

Then two older women, looking at her as she stands on the seat and nearly falls against the window because she's jumping up and down on a busy train, shake their heads. One says something about children in the rush hour. It is rush hour now. I am not an aggresive person, but after five hours on a train and their five-minute judgement of me and my family, I imagine grabbing their hair in my hands and pulling them kicking and screaming out of the train, opening their briefcases and

404

throwing the entire contents on the tracks and watching as the train mashes up whatever hideously important documents they are carrying. I get out the next picnic item. We have lychees, satsumas, BabyBel cheese. Any food that needs to be unwrapped, basically, and therefore takes up time on the journey.

I love getting the train with her. If it's well organised, she's the best companion in the world. If it's not well organised, I try to make cups into rockets a lot.

On the Train with a Toddler

There were tuts in her direction
that she didn't understand
as she strolled slowly from seat to seat
avoiding knees and sour looks she didn't see.

A sea of giants staring down at laptops
as she spun around between the seats
legs and hands and people
whose frowns she doesn't fully understand yet

because she loves the train
she loves the walk
she loves to talk to people
who after tiring days at work
in places they'd love to stay away from
wish she wasn't there.
Wish she wasn't trying to walk past them
or brush their knees by accident
or stare, smiling
Wish she wasn't trying to chat

or ask them nicely
if they want imaginary ice-cream
from her shop.

And sometimes when she stops at them
and smiles at them
and says hello
they stare down at their papers
scared she will not let them go
if they reply.

And when she asks me why they do not speak
I weakly tell her that
Some people travelling on the train just want some peace on
    their way back
because they've worked all day and do not want a kid walking
    quietly past their knees or trying to play with them or
    trying to say hello or sell them ice-cream made of air
    because they do not have the time for that

But I'm starting slowly to change my mind now

because when she asks me why she cannot smile
and try to chat and laugh and stare
after ten explanations that don't go anywhere
I tell her that she can.
You can.
Smile away, I say

'Cos this is your train
as much as theirs
and if you're walking slowly down the gangway

and anybody tuts and frowns
just turn around and tell them
what you tell me:

That you love the train
and love to walk
and love to smile
and love to talk
and nobody is getting hurt
and if your day at work was shit
and now you see a little kid
strolling down the gangway
not in anybody's way
just say hello for goodness' sake
it's not difficult to ask her how she's doing.
because she loves the train and loves to speak and play with
        other humans.

I tell her she's the normal one
she's the good example

I'm confusing her I think
but she just smiles and turns around
and as we pull up to King's Cross Station
she's excited
singing 'London Bridge is Falling Down'
not loud 'cos I won't let her
but still the frowns drown out my day
and when after the second verse someone whispers
in that very English way
not complaining to your face
just loud enough for you to hear the scowl

'Imagine parents bringing kids on trains in bloody rush
        hour.'

I bite my tongue again
but I am desperate to say:
that you do not own this time of day
this train or vital public space
it isn't just for business people
moody-faced and sour

and if you think for one split second that
I want to travel rush hour
with a toddler
then you are fucking mad
and there is not one carer, mum or dad I know that does.

But sometimes we must

So instead of frowning and moving knees away
whenever she is near
perhaps try to remember that
I do not want to be here either
trying to entertain a kid
in a train packed full of moody faces
teaching her that talking, walking, smiling
in these places
is a pain

because her brain is like a sponge
and the train is what she loves to travel on

where she can walk and chat and pull the tray back
picnic snacks and toddler rucksacks
packed with pens and paper
and distractions I have made her
so she won't get in your goddamn way
and won't make any goddamn noise
so you do not roll your goddamn tired working eyes at us

but I am tired too
more tired than you I think

as I try to smile and play and keep her safe
and out of everybody's way
on only two hours' sleep a night
for the last twenty-something days
but
like her

I love the train
I need the train
I love the way she plays
and packs her little bag excitedly
and squeals as it comes into view
and holds my hand and squeezes it
and jumps the gap and chooses where we'll sit
and eats the picnics that I always make

and sometimes she might cry
or occasionally shout
when she sees a sheep out of the window
or brush your knees by accident
or sing a bit too loud

and I'll do everything to keep the noise down
as we move from A to B
but she is only almost three and you,
you are fully grown
and she might be a nuisance as she says hello
but you are more of a pain to me and her
than you will ever know

for a little kid who is simply trying to say hello

14 NOVEMBER

2 years 8 months

I'm on the train again. Waving goodbye to Dee and Little One at the station is a bit heartbreaking sometimes but I'm only going for three days and I know they both love a few days without me there. It's great. Fish and chips, films and daddy nights. All good, so I'm not sure why I'm in tears.

It's Hard to Be Apart

We were one person at one time
Nine months you were inside
My blood ran through your system
My body fed your mind

And when you came out it was great
To hold your hand, to kiss your face
But despite the heavy pains
Sometimes I wish we'd stayed the same

'Cos now I watch you walk away
A little step more every day

My brain and eyes in constant game
To follow every move you make

To make sure you do not fall
Run too far and I can't call
And time passes too fast now
And though I love to see
You grow

It's so damn hard to be apart
My heart was pumping through your heart
We were one person at one time
I could protect you with my life

Sometimes I break down and cry
Just watching you stand by my side
And as the train pulls away
I just long to kiss your face

It's a love I can't describe
I will protect you with my life
And it's still hard to realise
At one time you were inside
And your blood flowed out of mine.

16 DECEMBER

2 years 9 months

The government has just announced a joint scheme to offer clothes vouchers in return for mothers to continue breastfeeding. Says it could encourage mums to carry on, the main point being that it could save the NHS millions if babies were breastfed longer. They're trialling it up in the north of England now. I was asked my thoughts on it. So I wrote about it. It's too long for a poem, a rant more, and perhaps I'll change my mind tomorrow but, well, I'm still a little gobsmacked they're even trialling this as an idea. It's brought back lots of feeding memories, good, bad and in between. Can't believe it's only nine months since the last feed. So odd. Well, not as odd as giving clothes vouchers to mums if they carry on breastfeeding though. What the hell do the government imagine breastfeeding is like? That easy, that a quick voucher will change your mind? Some of them must have done it, surely? Or at least seen their partners doing it?

Free Clothes Vouchers

Google images of breastfeeding
pick up magazines and parent books
and the mothers and the babies
seem to have the one same photoshoot:

413

Beautiful mum gazes at baby, blue veins photoshopped from
     boobs it seems
A house that looks like the stylist was from *Country Living*
     magazine

A tidy room.
Expensive rocking chair.
White shirt, white vest top,
Long blonde hair.
White cushions propped on bed or sofa
Twenty-eight or maybe older.
Mother smiles down lovingly.
She's pretty. Light-skinned, generally
Alone and close with looks of glee.
Baby latched on properly.

It's easy.
See.
It's lovely.
It's the best thing you can do.
For the baby and for you.
In calm-lit rooms.
Skin on skin.
Baby fed and soothed.

And I'm not saying that this can't be true.
Or that I don't think boobs are god
Or that I didn't love those moments
I'm just tired of these shots

These photo shots, this photoshopped
where no one moves and no one sobs

and I'm tired of never seeing that
and I can't afford those rocking chairs
'cos there's no space in our flat.
and I longed for a feeding chair
and not an aching back
and most days that I was feeding
I did not look like that –
I looked like crap!

Where are the babies with cradle cap?
Where are the stains on the mothers' clothes?
Where is the sick on their shoulders?
Why is she always happy she's alone?
Why is every mum feeding sitting on her own?
Where are the visitors or friends around?
Why does she never have to leave her house?
Where is the baby screaming out for more?
Why is no one ever tired or sore?
as bloodshot red eyes stare to space
'cos she's been up all night and up all day
as she tries to work out why her baby's crying once again.

Where are the real things mothers think about?
Staying home, scared to go out?
Worried where she might feed
Why do the photo'd nipples never bleed
cracked swollen and sore
Mastitis and cramping
babies trying to latch on but nothing is happening
Where are those moments when not everything's happy?
Where are the moments of guilt, anger and panicking?
Are we not allowed to talk about those?

So when I hear the word 'clothes'
Free clothes for free feeders!
I wonder the effect it would have on those bleeders
those mastitis mothers I know
or the mothers of pre-terms
or those worried about breasts
or the issues of feeding
or the reaction of friends
or not having support
or the job they ought to go back to quite soon
or the partner who says that those are his boobs
or the ones who have tried and don't know what to do
or the ones that don't want to for so many reasons
I think we should talk about those.

But instead we give vouchers for clothes.
Instead we give vouchers for clothes.
Two-hundred-quid vouchers for clothes.
'To make breastfeeding normal'
'To give incentive to those
who don't want to feed and who need to be bribed'
'To tackle the breastfeeding social divide'
'To tackle the economic reasons'

But if the reason was cash
everyone would be breastfeeding
'cos it's free!

And if we want to make it 'normalised'
get babies breastfed on TV
get a character to breastfeed on *Coronation Street*
and if you want to support parents

spend the money on *supporting* them
or if you really want to bribe me
I can think of better things to spend it on
than clothes:

I'd suggest some
government
Free sleep vouchers
Hot cup of tea vouchers
Hold your baby and allow you five minutes to eat vouchers
Put up your feet vouchers
Nipple leak vouchers
Have a quick wee vouchers
Adult talk vouchers
When you're bored vouchers
Cabbage leaves vouchers
Help me please vouchers!
Don't tell me to leave the hospital without making sure I can
        feed vouchers.
Paternity or grandparent leave vouchers
So someone can hold her and I can go sleep vouchers
Breathe vouchers
Or scream vouchers
When someone harasses me in town when I feed vouchers
A locked room
By myself
Just to weep vouchers
I just want to sleep vouchers

But I could feed vouchers
And it was lovely
For me

I could feed vouchers.
My nipples didn't bleed vouchers
My baby didn't bite
I had a partner and a mum to help me overcome the lonely
      nights
I had people there to take my baby so I that could have a nap
I had no complications with a kid who couldn't latch.
And after six months I went back to work
and replaced my daytime feed with mash.
I found it hard but know I had it easy
I found it sore but nothing bad

So give me my clothes vouchers
and bugger all my friends who couldn't do that
So give me my clothes vouchers
and bugger all the mums who didn't do that
just 'cos they apparently didn't give a shit
but would have done it fine and easy
with a quick two hundred quid
of clothes.

Especially those from northern parts
Or those whose bank account is not as big
But just a little question before I go and spend all of this . . .

Will you come and help me on the bus?
Into town with all the bags?
Take my baby for a walk so I can browse the shopping
      racks?
And if my baby starts to cry
and I have to feed her in the shops
will you put your arm around my waist

if someone stops and makes a fuss?
Or help me find the feeding room that often smells of wee?

So give me my vouchers now
and I'll go and buy some clean white clothes
to replace the ones with sick stains on
or milky nipple-leaking holes
that yellow-stain my feeding bras
and I'm sure there's loads of research about
why this plan might work
but to me it's just a farce

I find it rude
I find it classist
I find it weird
I find it wrong

We don't need clothes vouchers
We need support
We need feeding chairs for everyone
with clean white cushions on.

2 years 9 months

A pregnant woman wearing a niqab in Paris was attacked this month and put in hospital, where she lost her baby. Disgusting. Tragic. I am a bit late with all news at the moment. I read articles about banning the niqab in the UK. I keep thinking of the woman at toddler group who gets talked about constantly as she sits and looks after her beautiful wee boy.

It's getting colder now. All our kids are getting snotty.

Snotty Noses

The niqab covered her hair
We both stared at our kids
Snotty-nosed in the park
We both forgot tissues

I called my kid over
And wiped her nose with my sleeve
Pretty disgusting to do
But at least she could breathe

She called her kid over
And wiped off the snot

On the hem of her niqab
The kid trotted off

We laughed to ourselves
And checked no one would know
That we both had dry snot trails
Marking our clothes.

I wish there could be a headline in the paper about this, just for a bit
of balance:
Muslim Woman in Niqab Also Has a Child with a Snotty Nose!
or
Woman in Niqab Takes Son to Toddler Group
or
Woman in Niqab Feeds Son Water.

12 JANUARY

2 years 10 months

Oh shit. The questions have begun. This week they included:

Can Rapunzel build a bridge?

Is the world a jigsaw?

Are we made of bricks?

Why do we die?

I have a feeling I'm a bit out of my depth with this parenting malarkey now. I remember my dad telling me that traffic lights were controlled by very small people who sat inside them with three-colour torches. My friend's dad told her salt and vinegar crisps were made under the sea and that was why they were salty. We both believed them until we were nearly ten. I don't want to talk rubbish. If I don't know the answer to something I will say 'I don't know' and try to find out. Just as we are done potty training and I thought I could relax, pat myself on the back and have a cup of tea, now the philosophy course is starting. Kids should teach philosophy. I might tell her the traffic lights story though.

Answers:

If she learnt construction or engineering then, yes, I reckon no problem.

It depends how you look at it. It is made up of plates . . .

No. Do you want to share an ice-cream?

I don't know. Lots of people think different things, for example . . .

I'm Not Good at This

My daughter is nearly three
and she starts asking me about death

She said she didn't want to die
and didn't want me to die
and didn't want to look like Gran's friend
'cos she looked old and soon she'll die
and she asked me every day for months
why we die
and how we die
and I tried my best to answer her
but mostly I just cried.
I'm not good at these questions.

'Cos I cannot face the thought
and she told me not to worry
and that made me cry some more
and she said 'I love you Mummy'
and that made me cry till I was sore
and then she cuddled me
and walked away
and told me she was bored.
I'm not good at these sorts of questions.

But she kept asking me that night
and I tried my best to hold it down
told her flowers bloom then leaves fall
autumn orange turns to brown
I explained how winter comes with death
and all the leaves soak to the ground

She turned around and asked
if my granddad would come back in spring.
I'm not good at answering these things.

But my friend Lj told me
to be open about death
and I trust her and I've tried
I said I think my granddad's in the sky
that bodies decompose
but I don't know what happens to our minds

She asked me why she cannot fly
She asked me why she had to die
She asked me how and what and why
and when I said I didn't know
she asked me where we go
and I told her the same line –
I said 'We'll just have to have adventures
every day that we're alive'
that 'no one really knows quite why'
that 'some believe in God or gods'
that 'some believe you swap
your body for another thing'

She said she doesn't want to die
but when she does
she'll swap hers
with a fairy queen
and I can be her pet

She smiled and made me shake on it
Reincarnation it is!
She hasn't asked me anything
about death since.

I'm not very good at answering these questions.

27 JANUARY

2 years 10 months

This month I got an Arts Council grant of £6000 to work on putting together all the poems I've written about being a parent. Into a play. Or a monologue. Or something that I can actually do 'cos theatre is not really one of them. Thanks to Battersea Arts Centre and an amazing producer, Sophie Bradey, I can now quit my day job. I mean, I am actually going to quit. In real life. It's so heart-warming when someone believes in you like that. Just asks you if you fancy doing something. Helps you with the application. And it worked. Bloody aida! Focus on poetry. Be a poet. That sounds too wanky, my dad will laugh at that. Full-time poet. Damn. It doesn't sound very practical. I can't believe I can actually try to do poetry full time. God knows if it'll work out, but if I don't try . . .

2 years 11 months

It's a beautiful sight to see: picking Little One up at six p.m. after a day with Granddad. A full day, nine a.m. to six p.m. I slightly forced it. Totally forced it, in fact. Made sure Mum was working and Dee was away. Got a gig in Bristol so I'd go through Reading and Dad would be the single option for me being able to do the show. Because I can't wait any longer. She loves seeing him, he doesn't like the drive to us and I know he's astounding with kids. If I'm there, she wants me. If Mum's there, she wants 'Nanny'. So I hatched a plan. Dad alone with the child.

I'm not trying to be mean. I just want him to have a great relationship with her, like I did with my granddads. I realise that my dad is pretty petrified of looking after her – it's less lazy-fart syndrome, which I'd first thought, and more 'How the hell do I look after a kid on my own?' syndrome. The same way I felt when Dee went back to work after paternity leave. I was totally petrified of doing something wrong and harming a small person. I just assumed because Dad was, well, Dad, that he'd be fine with kids. He never said, 'To be honest, Hollie, I never looked after you on your own when you were little, I have no sodding idea how to change a nappy and am petrified she will choke or fall or run away from me and I will lose your child for ever if I have full responsibility.' If he'd said that, I would've got it. But I guess some men aren't really brought up to say, 'Help! I'm not able to do this! I've not done this before! I'm fucking scared!' Not this man, anyway. So

427

he just made jokes as always: 'I'm not changing a bloody nappy, that's for women', 'Wait till she's potty-trained', 'I'll get your mum to do it.'

So I had to properly plan. And it worked.

I ring the bell. Dad answers the door and I see him and Little One standing next to each other laughing. I make a cup of tea and sit down and listen for about half an hour as my dad doesn't shut up telling me all the things they've done, and how I have to tell her not to try to play hide-and-seek in the supermarket, and, did I know, she's really good with climbing, and did I know she can get to the swing by herself and did I know ... ?

Yes Dad, of course I fucking know these things. I've been with her pretty much every day for the first three years of her life. You'd know that too if ...

But I don't say that. Or think it, really. I'm just really bloody happy that it went well. Project 'Babysitter Number Three' is now complete. Otherwise known as Project 'I love you Dad, so does Little One, you are totally capable of being on your own with a child'. I've never seen my dad look so knackered, either. Tonight is the first time I've known him to go to bed before eleven p.m. in all my life. He actually said 'Sorry Hollie, I have to sleep, she never stops.' You don't say!

Omelette Pie

Since I was a kid
you've been telling me of work
of software and computing
and how important these things were
about your management
your company
the systems you controlled
and I remember your frustration
when I'd laugh and roll my eyes,

428

like
Yeah, yeah Dad.

It didn't mean I wasn't grateful
for the money that you made
for the detached house
my own bedroom
the yearly holiday
but I didn't get excited
about the business brain you have
because that's nothing to do
with my relationship to 'Dad'

Not your software I remember
but the hot chocolate machine
you'd let us use if we were careful
plastic cups filled up for free
and in work I'm sure you did a lot
but that's not who you are to me

You are Yahtzee games
and omelettes stuffed with
burgers, chips and peas
Burns Nights and
homemade cakes and
obsessions with cream tea
helping with my maths homework
or doing it for me
You are mince and mash
and treacle scones
and hockey club
and going on about

the shipyards every fucking time
we passed them on the way to Gran's
'where I worked as a lad'
'Yes Dad' we'd sigh
and roll our eyes again, us
'cheeky bastards in the back'

You are a family of grocers
your home bananas always black
you are stocking shelves after school
with sanitary pads
You are locking up
and going back
to check the doors one hundred times
calming me at Cambridge
and being there to give advice

So no matter how important
or good you were at work
that role will never be as key for me
as who you are with me
and her –
as the fact you spent the whole day
chasing her through parks
and that when I come to pick her up
she looks at you
and smiles and laughs
holds your hand
and hugs you
gives your cheeks a pat
then turns around and asks me
when she's coming back

So you can talk systems till your deathbed
and I'll still laugh and roll my eyes
because I'd really much prefer it
if you'd make your famous omelette pie
filled with chips and peas and burgers
for Little One to try
so she can save that in her memory
the way it's firmly stuck in mine.

2 years 11 months

After nearly three years I'm slowly realising that other people are not always right about parenting, and that maybe, just maybe, I should trust my instinct a bit. Not worry about others' opinions too much and just get on with it. Since I was pregnant, me and Dee have kept on being told to get a bigger house, change jobs, get our own garden, get married, get a car each, get into more of a routine, stop taking her to festivals or theatres or work in general. I've been stressing that we're doing it all wrong because of this. Then I look at her. She's healthy and happy. I'm done with all the judgement. I'll let her judge our parenting skills from now on. If she smiles, I'll take that as a pass. If she laughs, a straight A for us both.

OK, Mum

When I was pregnant, I was told to cover up
offered pretend rings for my finger
so I didn't just look 'knocked up'
baggy clothes to hide the 'lump'
and phrases used that made me want to vomit up
    again

On top of morning sickness
they said:
Do you really want a bastard child?
Do you really want a confused child?
Selfish woman with no ring
Think of your child's suffering!
Just get married, it's good for tax
You don't look pregnant, you just look fat
And when we went for lunch together:
A ringed finger just looks better.
They said *unmarried girls are tasteless*
and chaste despite our years
together
and whether I feel the same or not
I need to tie that knot
So I do not confuse my unborn child.
How will she understand why
you are not her daddy's wife?
I smiled, went to the flat and cried

wondering if the worry was all justified
and if I was making
a huge confusing
mess.

Now my child is all grown up
and when she asked about
the prince and princess
and why me and Daddy were not wed
I said we showed our love in others ways –
Made you, I say

She said *OK, Mum*
smiled
and walked away
to play with trains.

2 MARCH

Nearly 3 years old

I am so much better with toddlers than babies. I don't mean I'm amazing with toddlers, just better. I still have no desire to hold new babies. I feel really silly about this, like a total fraud. Lots of my friends are starting to have babies now and I think they expect me to be a 'baby person', 'cos I had one at one point a few years back.

I went to a friend's house to see her new baby last week. Loads of us were there and everyone was asking for a hold and a wee cuddle and I just forgot to ask. Dee asked. He always does, he's amazing with babies. But I just sort of forgot. I've been told loads that especially when your own kid grows up, you'll love looking at and holding and smelling babies and want to have another one of your own and feel all gooey and sad that your baby is no longer as small. It hasn't happened to me yet. I like them, I mean. I love babies as the small, innocent, beautiful human beings that they are, and I'll hold them till the planets collide in order to give the parents a rest. Not as much as Dee. He's like a professional party baby-carrier. But I just forget to ask, if it's just for a 'wee hug' rather than a saving swoop to ease that new mum 'I love my baby but don't want to hold it any more' hopeful glare. Dee nudged me at my friend's house to remind me to ask for a hold. It's a bit of a deal we have. But when I asked, I just sounded fake. 'Oooh, can I have a wee hold?' I said, hoping that it sounded like I genuinely wanted to, as Dee laughed into his drink.

It's the same way I feel about wedding dresses. I mean, I like them and I'll go shopping for them and I get really, really excited when my friends are happy and in love and trying on loads of beautiful gowns. But I don't get any overwhelming gushing feeling about the dresses themselves. I try to force myself into full hearty passionate excitement about these things, but it doesn't happen. I say 'That's beautiful' and stuff, because it is. I do mean it. But I always feel a bit like an actress. A bad actress. I cry at every wedding still though.

I especially hate it when people ask me 'Would you like a little hold?' and I look up as if it's a genuine question and I'm allowed to say, 'Nah, I'm all right with this alcoholic drink I can now down again', whilst realising I should have already asked to hold the new baby anyway. If you're *asked* if you want a hold, that means you have failed in your 'friend of the friend who's had a new baby' role. You should never have to be asked. That's bad.

So I hold babies and look at their sweet faces and think about how the world needs to get better for them and how we should stop buying so many shit plastic toys and plastic party bags filled with smaller shit plastic toys that are in our plastic bins within a week and plastic bottles of water that will ravage their drinking sources as they grow up and more and more fishermen will be trying to support their families by fishing for plastic bottles from polluted rivers because there are no more living fish left. That makes my heart beat faster. In panic. I panic when I look at babies. I panic when I hold them. Babies make me a bit sad. We need to step our game up for them.

Plastic Bottles

There's not much I find as backward
as plastic bottles filling shores

There's not much for me that sums up
why less is often more
than fresh water
wrapped in plastic
making money
sold and branded

There's not much I find as pointless
as plastic bottles filling shores

Water packaged and sold back to us,
now polluting its own source

So I think about plastic a lot – not enough still though. But I don't smell babies much. And I don't feel too nostalgic, I mainly think 'It's nice I don't still have a baby, that was fucking hard work', and look lovingly at my nearly three-year-old before I hand the small, beautiful bundle of joy to someone else so I can grab a drink and chat with my child about why she can't have another sip of beer. I don't like feeling nostalgic. She's lush as she is. Especially now we can have a drink together!

I love that children get a sense of humour so fast and that, even by two years old, we can geek out together about words. I love this new side of motherhood that's panning out as she grows up. It makes my heart tingle in thrills the same way translation exams and maths puzzles do when I realise my kid seems as geeky as me.

Yesterday we were playing nurses where Little One is the nurse and I am a patient who lies on the floor with my eyes closed and feet on the 'hospital cushion' and gets a check-up that lasts as long as I can draw it out. My friend Juliet taught me this game. I saw her lying down on the couch as her daughter and mine inspected her feet for ten minutes. She's a legend in general, even more so for introducing Little One to a love of this 'Mum is the patient' scenario. It's pretty much a free foot massage.

Anyhow, we were playing this brilliant game. Little One told me that the teddy needed a check-up. I said 'She'll just have to be patient', at which point Little One screamed and started running around the room full pelt in manic circles.

'Mum! Mum!'

Laughing hysterically and almost passing out with all the racing about:

'Mum! There are two patients! "Patient" when you're waiting and "patient" when you're at the doctor's. Teddy has to be a patient patient!'

Another three minutes' sprinting around the room screaming 'Patient patient!', and she still wasn't over it. That's the shit right there that I fucking love – homonyms. Babies don't give a shit about homonyms.

'Patient patient.' If that doesn't excite you more than the smell of a new baby . . .

Very nearly 3 years old

OK, so maybe sometimes I feel a little nostalgic. Only sometimes, mainly late at night. It still amazes me how impressive boobs are. Even if it is the middle of the night, pitch-black, and I stumble into Little One's room if she's crying, and even if she's fast asleep and just calling out in her dreams, her hand still manages to shoot out of the covers, grab my boob, and then she's fine. Totally cool. A quick grope and she's back in the land of nod. I wish the boob thing had never freaked me out, 'cos really, it is pretty bloody amazing how much these parts of my body can do for one small being. I've never realised it before, but as well as the whole milk and calming nipple thing, they really are brilliantly warm, soft, and full of heartbeats. We *should* be bloody obsessed with them.

My Chest

You fed every two hours the month you were born
By two months you fed every four
At six months old I worked three days a week
Fed either end with mashed food in between
By the time you were one it was just twice a day
Before bed and at five a.m. so you slept until eight

By one and a half just once when you wake
At two you just ate food from a plate
Now you're almost three, eating soup, fruit and veg
But still put your palm on my chest when you're stressed
As the warmth and the beat of my blood makes you calm
You lay your cheek to sleep, on my heart.

3 years old

I'm on the plane back from the Cúirt Literature Festival in Galway. It was such a brilliant festival. And Galway is totally magic. I forgot my words once but apart from that, all good. I'm on the plane surrounded by adverts and promotions and newspapers and people complaining about Ryanair, the low-cost airline. A woman in the check-in queue spent the entire time telling me why she hates Ryanair. People always complain about Ryanair while they are taking a Ryanair flight.

Little One woke every two hours the night before I flew to Galway. She was being sick all night and I felt awful doing this trip. FaceTime is helpful now, and I love seeing her and Dee's faces smiling at me through cyberspace. I'm knackered today – Ireland is always great to go to, but for some reason I can never just do the gig and go back to the hotel. The parties are always better here. And perhaps 'cos I'm further from home I feel freer and more excited, and more likely to be dancing till my eyes remind me I've got a child that is going to keep me awake the whole next day. So I need to try to sleep now.

I'd love a cup of tea if the steward would come. I look out of the window and realise the sun is setting and the clouds outside look like giant bright satsuma marshmallow fields and I hadn't even noticed because I'd been so busy getting annoyed about the adverts and the uncomfy seats and the people complaining about Ryanair. But I can't stop looking out of the window now. The world is so damn beautiful when you're above the clouds. Even on a packed Ryanair plane.

It's such a treat to be up here. It's such a treat to go to a festival in Ireland and see new places and meet new people. I miss her, though. But I love getting away for a couple of days. It just makes going back to her so much better. I always feel romantic about motherhood when I'm not at home! Not checking for poo, or trying to be patient so she can put her shoes on herself and I stand clenching my teeth and holding my hands back from helping because we're going to be late again and I just want to rush her but know she'll never learn to do things herself that way. But when I'm away, those things seem funny and lovely and sweet. I love her so much. The sky is unreal. The clouds are snow peaches. If I hold my fingers round my eyes like binoculars so I can't see the window edges it all looks like thick, beautiful peachy snow. The tea is here.

Ryanair: The Space above the Clouds

My daughter's face is like the space above the clouds
vast, searching, untouched
wise and earthly
painfully truthful
and so so beautiful
sometimes I don't know what to do when I look at her

I spy stars in her dimples as she smiles
and a tiny line deepening between her eyes
etching life into her skin as she thinks

I watch out of the window
wondering what the next sunset will bring her
as I sink into my seat

Orange stripes stretched in front of me
waiting for the steward to offer me a tea
that tastes like tar, I'm sure

I wonder what she'd think if she were here with me
far above the mapped-out lights below
staring out of the window
watching as the world runs away
slow motion from the sun again
as clouds layer the sky like soft Antarctic ice
and darken to a fuzz of rainbow shades
and the air fades from white and blue to red
orange, yellow, pink and black again

I wonder what she'd think of that
I wonder how many lines this sunset
would carve into her skin
I wonder where the thought lines
and the smile lines would begin
if I told her things my dad told me
like how it cannot rain in the space above the clouds
and how outer space is the only space above us now
and how the plane is racing the earth as it turns around
never stopping for a cuppa

As the day turns into dusk in front of us
I look up at the moon
thank the man
and sip my tea
it tastes like tar
but the window view is heavenly

I hope she's looking at the stars right now
but Dad is doing bedtime
so there's no way she'll be awake

She is three soon and she is happy
and sometimes I need to remember
to feel less guilty and more proud

I wave behind the window from the space above the clouds
in case she's looking at me now

looking down on cities and the houses lining towns
all the people buzzing round
struggling
thinking they are doing
so much worse than all the rest

We are a dust speck in this universe
She is probably asleep
I close my eyes and sip my tea
it tastes like tar
but the window view is sweet enough

I try to find the stars
as the glowing sky fades into black

I can't wait to kiss her forehead
as she sleeps
when I get back

14

SPRING
THREE YEARS OLD

14 APRIL

You are three years old. You really are starting pre-school. Your clothes are neat, face scrubbed clean and your hair slicked back smartly in a twisting ponytail like only Dee can do. You are ready for the classroom. I'm not sure how that happened.

'Bye Mum.'

You seemed less bothered than me.

I sit in a café and read for three hours. I have been waiting for this for a while. I promised myself months back that when this moment came I would not use the time to go home and work or clean or cook or anything that I've been managing to fit in so far in the minimal time I've had. No, I would spend the three hours doing something else. Something for me, something I've not had the time to do any more since having a child. I go to the park and read a magazine from cover to cover. It's amazing.

The time flies past. I go and pick you up and you smile, running out of school. I am a mum standing outside a school collecting my kid. It is a bit surreal. I am actually a mum. Properly. Your smile is magical. You were OK. I am so relieved.

Me: 'So, how was pre-school? Was it great? Was it great fun?' (leading questions)

Little One: 'Yes it was Mum, it was really fun.'

Me: 'That's so so great, oh I'm so happy.'

And I am. We hold hands and start slowly tottering home.

Little One: 'Yeah. But I don't think I'll go back again.'

And I realise I forgot to tell her it's not a one-off. I just assumed she'd know.

Damn.

I'm not very good at this.

ACKNOWLEDGEMENTS

I would never have thought about sharing these diaries or poems with anyone if it wasn't, first and foremost, for Dee. While I was jotting down thoughts on pregnancy, babies and all that, he was constantly saying 'you should record these – you should share them'. 'Nah,' I said, 'who wants to hear about this stuff?' I didn't think anyone would relate to them or give a toss – the opposite, in fact. So he pushed me into a recording studio, stuck headphones on my head and made me read ten of the poems I'd written before our daughter's first birthday into a mic. About six months later, after hundreds of downloads, he suggested I put a poem I wrote called 'Embarrassed' onto my YouTube channel. 'Nah,' I said, 'not that one, no one will relate to it.' He pestered me again. Then one night, I walked into the lounge and the video camera was set up 'just in case'. After that poem was shared online about a million times by parents, midwives, nurses, doulas, baby groups, parenting websites and, well, people, I realised perhaps he had a point; perhaps I wasn't the only one feeling how I felt.

So thanks to you for pushing me to do this, this book, and the whole poetry malarkey in general, despite the potential embarrassment of being written about. You are an angel for sure. You'll realise one day perhaps. Thanks also for being the most excellent support, partner and father imaginable.

Thanks to our two mums for giving birth to us (well done) and for being such excellent new grandmas – I would've likely broken down without your help – and to my mum for all of your trips and advice, and, well, everything. Thanks to the two granddads for taking credit for the grandmas' work and then coming into their own as granddads a bit later on! To all our supportive family and great friends and to the NHS and all their brilliant midwives.

As important . . . thanks to all of those people who have read or listened or shared my writing further and wider than I would ever have done myself. Thanks to all of those lovely jubbs who have replied to haters on YouTube so quickly that I've not had to do it myself and to anyone who has ever come to a gig, supported a gig, shared a poem or organised an event I was at. A bit like parenting, the poetry world seems to rely on a lot of enthusiastic people doing a lot of work for free. Thanks to my favourite poetry nights for asking me to come and complain into a microphone – too many to mention, though for this book specifically – Bang Said the Gun (first place I read 'Embarrassed' live), Shambala Festival (first place I read an extract from this book), and the ABM (Association of Breastfeeding Mothers) and Breastfeeding Festival for being so nice about my writing.

To the huge support of superproducer Sophie Bradey for your belief in these stories despite my inability to do theatre with them, to Battersea Arts Centre, the Arts Council and the Arts Foundation Award (and Neneh Cherry for sticking up for the motherhood theme), without which I would never have had the time or money to write this all out and work and be a parent at the same time. No chance. And to Luke Wright for his advice to 'just go with the women wave for a while' when I was worried about the one-sidedness of my writing.

To Becky Thomas for hauling her stiletto-heeled beauty around to get this published and Rhiannon Smith and Little, Brown for thinking that people may possibly want to read this stuff. I'm still unsure. So is my mum. (Love you Mum!)

Lastly, to my Gaga, Papa, Gran and Grandad for being the most lovely grandparents with the most brilliant stories I could've wished for.

And Gaga – please excuse my bad language, but as you've said before: 'If anyone has the right to swear, it's a mother.'

INDEX OF POEMS